SPORT HORSE

SOUNDNESS AND PERFORMANCE

DEDICATION

This English edition is dedicated to the memory of Dr Kieran Bredin MRCVS, 1938–2003, an expert equine surgeon, horse friend and a gentleman, who kindly – and at an unexpected time – encouraged my childhood ambition of going to vet school.

SPORT HORSE

SOUNDNESS AND PERFORMANCE

TRAINING ADVICE for DRESSAGE, SHOWJUMPING and EVENT HORSES
by CHAMPION RIDERS, EQUINE SCIENTISTS and VETS

Dr Cecilia Lönnell

Foreword by George H. Morris

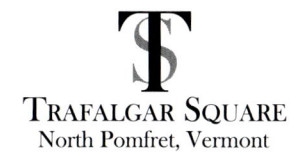

Trafalgar Square
North Pomfret, Vermont

First published in the United States of America in 2017
by Trafalgar Square Books North Pomfret, Vermont 05053

Originally published 2016 in Swedish as Träna Hästen För Framgång Och Hållbarhet

The right of Dr Cecilia Lönnell to be identified as the author of this work has been asserted in accordance with the Copyright, Design and Patent Act 1988

The information in this book is true and complete to the best of our knowledge. All recommendations are made without any guarantee on the part of the publisher. The author and publisher shall have neither liability nor responsibility to any person or entity with respect to any loss or damage caused or alleged to be caused directly or indirectly by the information contained in this book. All rights reserved. No part of this book may be reproduced or transmitted in any form or by any means, electronic or mechanical including photocopying, recording or by any information storage and retrieval system, without permission from the Publisher in writing.

Trafalgar Square Books encourages the use of approved riding helmets in all equestrian sports and activities.

ISBN: 978 1 57076 837 8
Library of Congress Control Number: 2017946803

Cover design: Sharyn Troughton
Book design: Anna Ågren and Sharyn Troughton

Photo research: Sofia Hannar, Dr Cecilia Lönnell
Photographs by Jon Stroud, Bob Langrish, Roland Thunholm (including front cover), Suzanne Fredriksson, Krister Lindh, Pelle Wahlgren and the author

Dr Peter Kallings, DVM provided expert advice on Chapter 11 *Supplements, medication and doping*

Printed in Malaysia

CONTENTS

Foreword		7
Acknowledgements		13
1.	**BACKGROUND – WHY THIS BOOK?**	16
2.	**THE HORSE'S BODY – ANATOMY AND FUNCTION**	32
	The internal organs	34
	The musculoskeletal system	37
3.	**PREVENTING INJURY**	46
	What does scientific research say?	48
	What do champion riders and top vets say?	56
4.	**THE 'RIGHT' HORSE – ARE YOU A GOOD MATCH?**	66
	Points to consider	68
	Are you a good match?	72
	Advice when buying a horse	81
5.	**ALLOW YOUR HORSE TIME**	82
	Show the young horse respect	85
	Treat the horse as an individual	86

6.	**YOUR RESPONSIBILITIES AS A RIDER**	**92**
	The horse's manager – you	**94**
	Improving yourself mentally and physically	**96**
	Build a skilled team	**112**
7.	**FEEDING, SUPPLEMENTS AND WATER**	**116**
8.	**RIDING SURFACES – VARY WHERE YOU RIDE**	**122**
	Surface characteristics and use	**125**
	Maintenance	**126**
9.	**TRAINING**	**128**
	Basic training principles	**130**
	Injury risk and training antidotes	**139**
	Training planning	**150**
10.	**COMPETITION PLANS AND TRAVEL**	**166**
	Competition planning	**168**
	Travelling (to competitions)	**170**
11.	**SUPPLEMENTS, MEDICATION AND DOPING**	**176**
	References – Scientific studies	**183**

FOREWORD
by George H. Morris

I've known Cecilia Lönnell for a long time, having shown extensively in Sweden and taught many, many clinics there over the years. I'm very fond of her and fond of that country. To be asked to participate in a book that also features such an illustrious young group of equestrian superstars is a great honour.

What Cecilia has done here is she's gone back to the past and at the same time shown how knowledge from solid experience is supported by modern equine veterinary research. Nothing here is new, and that, with horses, is always better. I never in my life spent in equestrian sport pretended to reinvent the wheel. I was a copier. I copied Bert de Némethy. I copied Gordon Wright as a teacher. I copied Bill Steinkraus. To this day my whole day is spent trying to understand old, classic principles. Be it teaching, be it riding, be it training, be it care of the horse – that is all I try to do, every day of my life. Gordon Wright used to say, 'Nothing is new, we just do it better and quicker than we used to.' And that's what we get from the best horsemen – it isn't new, it just might be better and quicker.

Here, Cecilia has encapsulated all the points it takes to produce a horse – be it a pleasure horse or an Olympic horse, it doesn't matter. The points laid out on these pages are about *what is best for the horse.* Often in competitive riding, in all disciplines, we go off on tangents that are contrary to the best interests of the horse. Artificial devices, artificial footing – this is not what's best for the horse.

When you talk about horses and you talk about horse sport as Cecilia is, your first consideration is the management of the horse. If you buy a Hickstead or an Azur and send him to a third-rate boarding house, in about two seconds, you're going to have a third-rate horse. The most important thing is what the great old Virginia horsewoman and trainer of Conrad Homfeld and Joe Fargis Frances Rowe used to call 'beautiful care': how the barn is set up, the bedding of the stall, the feed programme, the vet, the equine dentist, the farrier, the quality of the grooming – it all should be *beautiful care*. Many of the riders quoted in this book are more hands-on in terms of stable management than I ever was, but our mission is the same: to give our horses *beautiful care*.

The greatest horsemen in the world – and I'm not necessarily talking about riding here – are the English. They always have been. Now I'm not saying the French, the Germans, the Swedes, the Dutch aren't good horsemen – they're all great and each is different – but I've traveled just about every country in the world and as far as the care and management of the horse, the greatest horsemen in the world are the English. That's why all the continental riders get English grooms to take care of their horses – horse care is in their blood. Being an American from the Northeast part of the country, I grew up with an offshoot of English horsemanship, and the whole thing is based on *natural*: turning horses out, riding through the country. Carl Hester revolutionized dressage because he approached it from a technical, scientific point of view, but allowed his English horsemanship to take it to a different level. We all know he is, yes, a very talented rider, but what really 'woke up' the dressage world is that he hacks his horses out, turns his horses out, shows that dressage horses should not be circus animals confined in stalls. He, and many other contributors to this book, assert that this should be the standard.

Bert de Némethy, who was a Hungarian trained in Germany,

managed the US equestrian team beautifully during his tenure, and he always had us work our horses on different surfaces – something that Beezie Madden notes as key in this book and is also supported by scientists. We would base at Aachen and Bert would have us ride gymnastics on the turf fields (which are now some of the warm-up rings) but often we also rode in the old dressage ring where the footing was quite deep. I would cheat with my hot horses that were above the bit – I would get them on the bit by tiring them out in that deep sand. But we rode on the roads, we rode on the turf, we rode in sand. Today too many horses are always worked on the same artificial 'perfect' footing, as some call it.

After management of the horse, the next most important consideration is selection of a horse for his rider and for his 'job.' And this is just as applicable to a school horse as it is to Big Star. The school horse is just as valuable as Big Star. Actually, everyone knows there's nothing as valuable as a top school horse! Selecting the right horse for a particular rider and a particular job depends on a mix of experience and instinct – some people, even laymen who maybe aren't so experienced, they have an eye for a horse, whether the best fit for an amateur hunter rider, a top dressage rider, a Rolex eventer, whatever. The great thing about this book is that Cecilia has included this kind of information, and it is dispensed by individuals who are current, they are champions, people know them. They're not people like myself, out of the dark ages. Their advice is all very relevant, and they are all saying the same thing.

Next you get to my pet peeve: the way people ride their horses. The United States historically has always been very weak in dressage. It is an afterthought. In the early days we had Thoroughbred horses that were so courageous and so special that we fudged dressage. Now we've finally caught up, and England has caught up, but 'fudging dressage' is still haunting the world, because I go all over the world and people are faking it everywhere. Faking it and tying horses down is crippling horses. There was a great about-face five or six years ago because of *Rollkur*. Overflexing horses is very damaging to the horse, and luckily, it has taken a swing for the better. However, it is not good enough, especially in the jumpers –

event horses and dressage horses have to more or less stay to the correct line because they are judged, but jumpers, they just strap them down, tie them down, put this on them, that on them, and away they go. The sport community – jumpers, eventers, dressage riders, and I mean in every country – must address how we work the horse, that whatever the discipline, it should be according to classical principles. The dressage work for sport horses has been a weak link, probably throughout history. And it still is a weak link. And I will speak up about it. It's not rocket science. There are books hundreds of years old that tell you how to work a horse!

In addition to not fudging dressage, great riders don't overjump. The two cripplers of a horse are footing and jumping. Knowing this, all the great riders don't overjump. We work a horse every day for condition, for discipline, for rideability. A friend of mine, Peder Fredricson (a Swede), he works the horse beautifully, so I will pick him out. He works a horse without auxiliary reins, he's had a vast background in correct dressage, and I watched him at the Olympics in Rio de Janeiro, where his quality of work was rewarded as he won individual silver. I am closely aligned to Beezie Madden – I know she's not an overjumper. Laura Kraut is definitely not an overjumper. John Whitaker, my idol of all the people I've ever seen, since I started riding – he's my idol of idols – he hacks out, he walks on roads, he doesn't overjump his horses. I was a driller when I was young. I drilled horses and was a culprit of overjumping. That's how I know that overjumping is the kiss of the death. At best a horse gets stale, at worst he gets sore or lame.

These three important points – management, selection, and how we ride – are the topics Cecilia has pulled together in this book under the auspices of the superstars and scientists of today, giving old information credibility. And in some ways it's all old news…but it's forgotten news. Lots of young people today, they're so competition-oriented, they forgot the whole point. Horse show horse show horse show. Ranking ranking ranking. I wouldn't still be doing this sport the way I still do it, teaching and riding, if that was all it was. That is very, very limited. These 'desperate housewives' and 'weekend warriors,' as I call them, have not yet been influenced to understand the point. And *that* is the point of this book. When I was under the tutelage of Bert de Némethy, we were a very classy group of young guys – we could afford to live well. But we learned from him and our other trainers in those days, *the point* was the daily work, the dressage, the beautiful care. The horse show was just an occasional test that showed us where we were in relation to the other people; then we went home and took care of our horses, schooled our horses. But a lot of people at horse shows today, all over the world – it's not just one country – they've lost the plot of what this is about. It's not just about rankings, points, and selection for championships – that's the icing on the cake.

Cecilia has done a great service to the sport: What she has gathered here is so correct, all going back to the past, but couched in modern perspective. People say about me, 'Oh, he's old fashioned. The sport has passed him.' Well, the greatest compliment I can get as a horseman is that I'm old-fashioned. The sport has not passed me; there's nothing different about working a horse the classical way, about caring for him as suits his nature. The future is the past.

George H. Morris

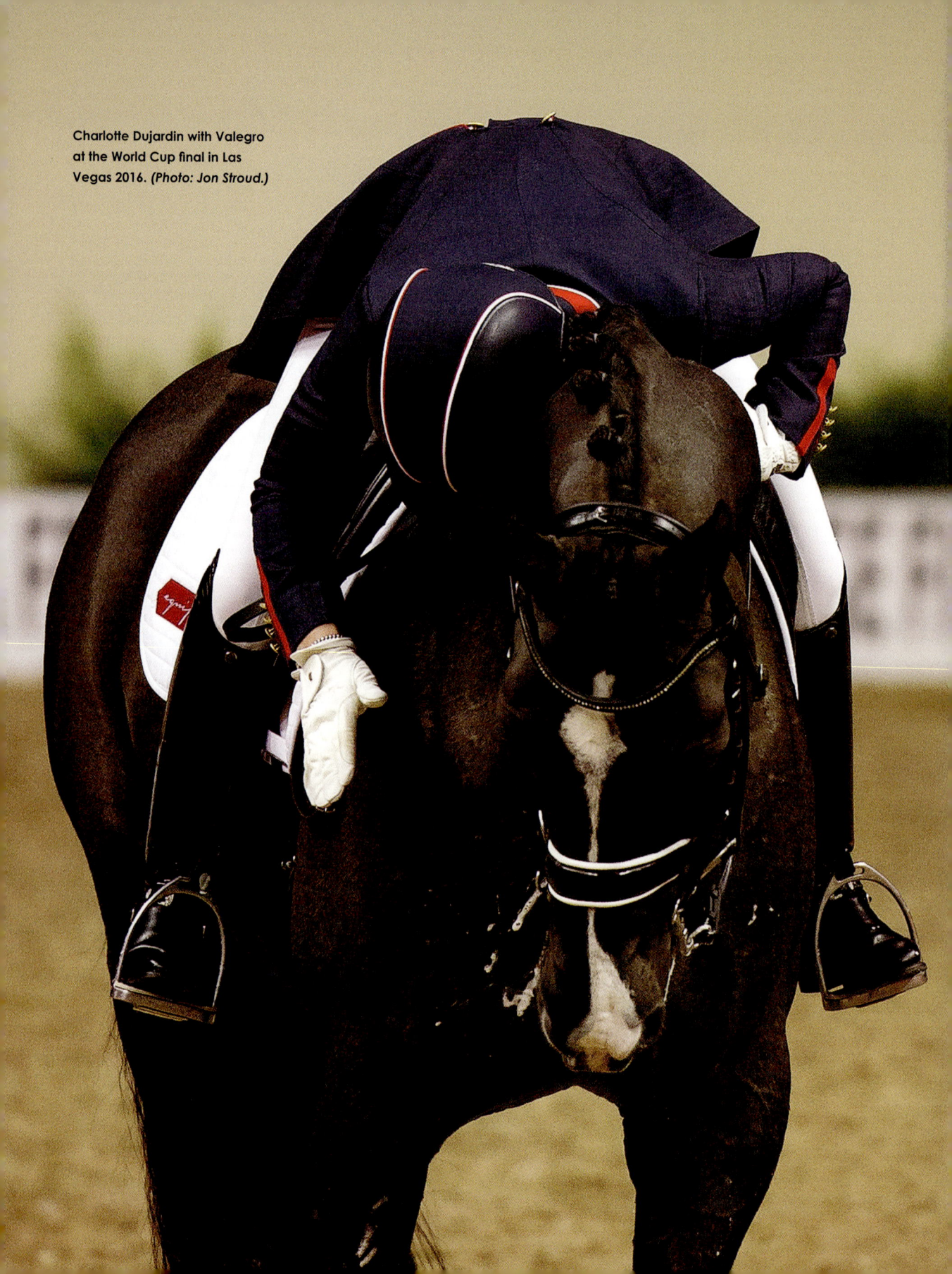

Charlotte Dujardin with Valegro at the World Cup final in Las Vegas 2016. *(Photo: Jon Stroud.)*

ACKNOWLEDGEMENTS
– *thank you!*

This book was some forty years in the making, and consequently there are very many people to whom I owe gratitude.

This English edition is entirely thanks to Andrew Johnston of Quiller Publishing, and was improved thanks to editor Martin Diggle. George Morris was extremely kind to take time to write the foreword, and I am in awe of the honour.

I am also very indebted to the champion riders and veterinary colleagues quoted, who have given up time for interviews and (for the riders), sometimes stable visits. Also, huge thanks to the elite riders in four countries who participated in the FEI-WHW study on training and equestrian surfaces quoted in this book. They, and members of their family or staff, very kindly put in a huge amount of work for the study to keep training diaries, answer questions, etc. A big thank you also to the staff of Swedish riding schools who participated in the riding school study (plus the insurance company AGRIA who gave access to its databases).

Working at the Royal Veterinary College in London was a privilege; massive thanks to my supervisors Professor Joanna Price, Professor Allen Goodship and Professor Dirk Pfeiffer.

The project at the Swedish University of Agricultural Sciences on injury risks in riding horses would not have been realised without my supervisors Professors Agneta Egenvall and Lars Roepstorff, Katarina Nostell and Johan Bröjer.

A huge thank you also to the research groups collaborating with our group in Uppsala on the European Footing and Training Study in the Netherlands, UK and Switzerland, led by Professor Rene van Weeren, Dr Rachel Murray and Professor Michael Weishaupt respectively, and to the International Equestrian Federation and World Horse Welfare who financed it. The FEI former first Vice-Presidents Sven Holmberg and John McEwen had key roles in this being realised. Other important grant sources for the research I have been engaged in have been The British Horse Betting Levy Board, the Swedish-Norwegian Foundation for Equine Research and the former Swedish Animal Protection Board.

I received support and great fellowship from my fellow Ph.D students and other colleagues, especially Dr Elin Hernlund, Dr Cecilia Wolff and Dr Karin Alvåsen at the Swedish University of Agricultural Sciences at Uppsala, Dr Brendan Jackson and Professor Kristien Verheyen at the Royal Veterinary College in London, and Carolyn Tranquille at the Animal Health Trust in Newmarket and Sofia Boqvist and Lisel Huse-Olsen, co-Erasmus students at the Veterinary Faculty in Utrecht, which started my interest in epidemiology. Dr James Wood at the Animal Health Trust and Dr Göran Dalin at Uppsala kindly paved the way for my coming to England after vet school.

The book would also not have happened without *Ridsport* magazine who, through the years, have kindly sent me to six equestrian Olympics and commissioned a majority of the interviews quoted, and in the early stage of the writing process kindly made their archives available. A big thank you also the Swedish equestrian magazines *Hippson, Häst & Ryttare, Kentaur* and *Showjumping* who also commissioned articles quoted in the book.

The book would certainly not have happened without the

encouragement of Mari Zetterqvist-Blokhuis, the publisher contact of Pether Markne, and my Swedish editor Erika Palmqvist. Herself a horse owner, she liked and improved the idea and encouraged me. Thanks also to Sofia Hannar and Anna Åhman, equally skilled at editing and design, who had the final roles of turning the Swedish typescript into a book, and to their UK colleagues Becky Bowyer and Sharyn Troughton, who handled this edition, plus Tiina Nevala at Massolit who made it possible at the Swedish end. I am also indebted to the photographers, Jon Stroud, Bob Langrish, Roland Thunholm, Suzanne Fredriksson, Krister Lindh and Pelle Wahlgren for their stunning pictures and to Professor Stina Ekman and Dr Fredrik Södersten and Professor Leo Jeffcott for permission to use their cartilage, tendon and bone images.

An important aid to the writing process came from 'test readers'; Eva Dahlberg, Dr Elin Hernlund, Suzanne Fredriksson, Sofie Wernborg and Anna Singer for the first draft and Marcus Lundholm, Åsa Stibner, Markuu Söderberg and Dr Sofie Viksten of the final version.

Finally, sincerest thanks to my late parents Curt and Birgitta and other family, and dear friends Philippa Kindersley in England, Louise and Ken Parkhill in Ireland and Annica Triberg-Håkansson in Sweden who, through their friendship, contacts, and support, set the whole process in motion a long time ago, and helped realise it.

With so many people having assisted me in the production of this book, I had better add a heartfelt apology to anyone I've inadvertently omitted to mention.

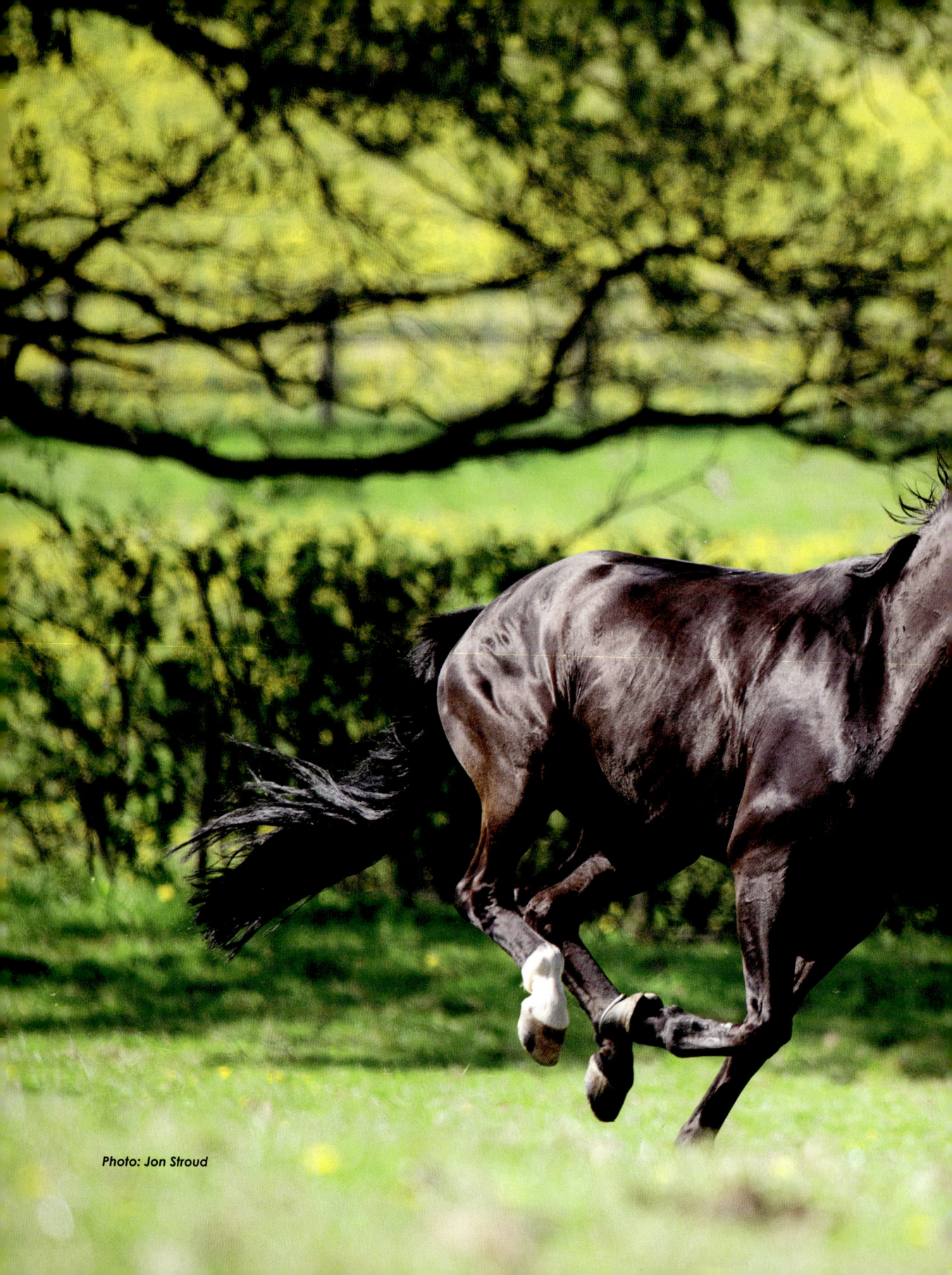

Photo: Jon Stroud

1. Background
– why this book?

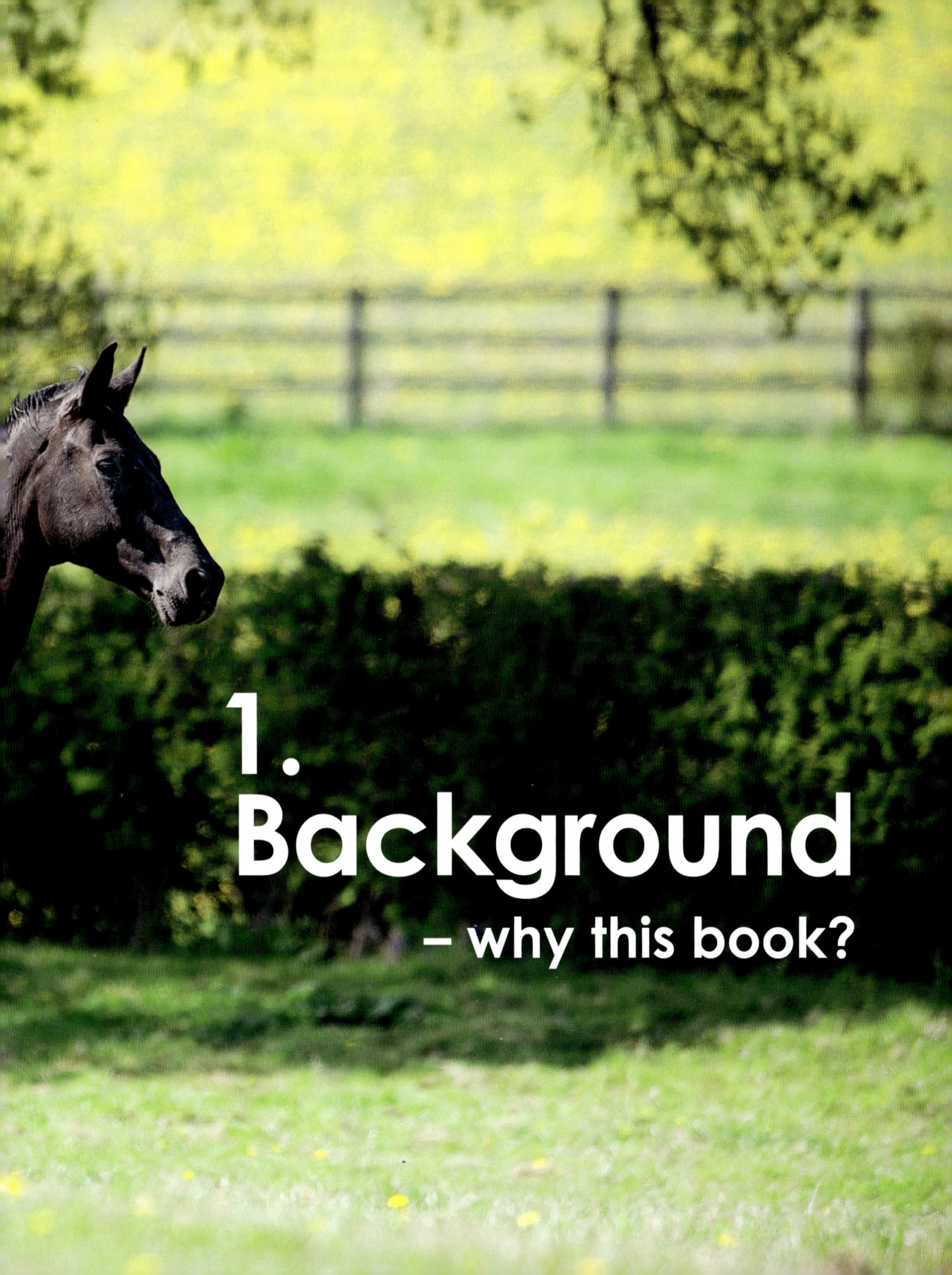

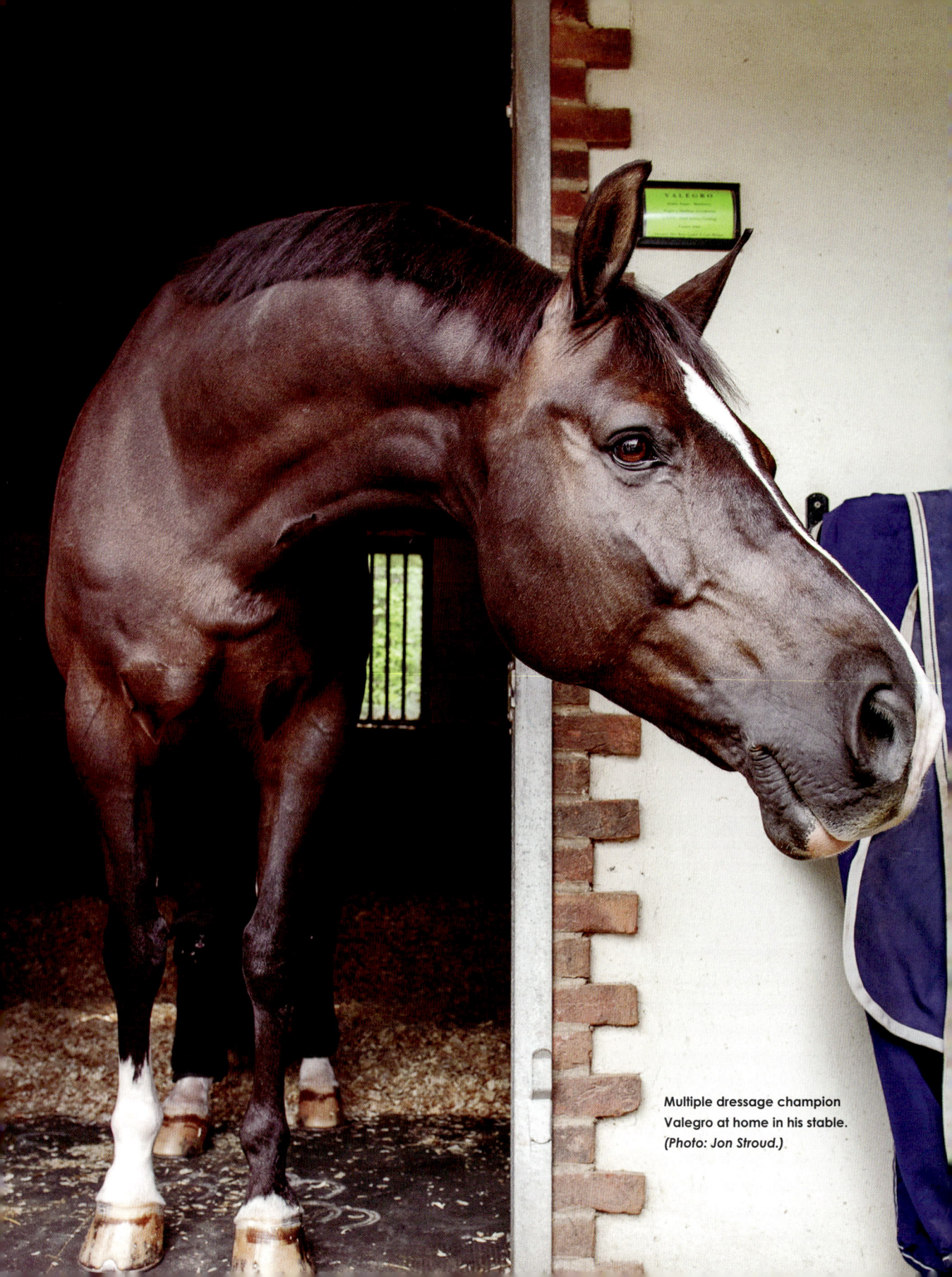

Multiple dressage champion Valegro at home in his stable. *(Photo: Jon Stroud.)*

BACKGROUND – WHY THIS BOOK?

So what is the key to success as a rider? Having had the privilege of following equestrian sport at top international level for over forty years one key observation can be divided into one piece of good news and one piece of bad news. The bad news is that there are few shortcuts to be had with horses. The only way to reach long-term success in riding is to have the best possible coach/teacher and to be surrounded by a good team, and to be prepared to put in your own hard work. The latter is the good news – that it is possible for a rider to go very far, all the way to the top of the world, by putting in a lot of hard work, striving to learn and paying attention to detail. This, rather than any 'silver bullet', is the secret behind almost all equestrian success. In the US, dressage star Laura Graves (the 2017 World Cup final silver medallist) is a recent example. Both she and Charlotte Dujardin started off doing stable work as working students. Whatever your level as a rider, the will to work hard, striving to learn and attention to detail will help you to improve and to win. It is, of course, true for most sports that it is impossible to reach the top without your own hard work.

Many books about riding are based on advice about how to make the horse perform what the rider wants, whether it is dressage movements or jumping fences, in the best possible way, in a arena or cross-country. This book is more focused on what you, as a rider, can do to make it easier for the horse to perform what you want, what is reasonable to demand from a particular horse at his current level of training, fitness and strength, and how you can develop that fitness and his motivation and confidence. A horse may be extremely well-bred and possess huge talent, but with inappropriate training, riding or management he and his rider runs the risk of having repeated setbacks and get few chances of winning.

Olympic team champion Laura Kraut has quoted a study

'As a rider you can go very far, all the way to the top of the world, by putting in a lot of hard work, striving to learn and paying attention to every little detail. (It is, of course, true for most sports that it is impossible to reach the top without your own hard work).'

'Keep the horse happy and give him as good a life as possible' says John Whitaker in his soundness advice later on in this book.

> 'As a rider you must think of the horse as a four-legged athlete and yourself as the manager.'
> **Ludger Beerbaum**

of the hallmarks of a champion showjumper, who has the scope to stay at the top over time. There are six points (the parenthesis are my own comments to Laura's list).

1. Riding talent (what that entails can be discussed for hours, but this list shows it is not the be-all and end-all of a rider's potential).
2. The will and ability to work hard (to develop experience and skills).
3. Robust personal health (necessary for that hard work).
4. Being mentally strong (to overcome setbacks, handle competition and other pressures and, again, work hard).
5. Social skills (not as in being the centre of the party but developing good relationships with horse owners, potential sponsors, other riders, and media).
6. The skill to keep your horse(s) sound and healthy (as again without that you will have few chances of winning and horse owners will lose heart).

How injuries develop in a horse – or a human athlete or fitness enthusiast – is a complicated process that is still far from fully investigated. Experts do, however, know that orthopaedic injuries arise from an interaction of internal and external factors such as genetics, conformation, upbringing, management and training. In horse sports, arena surfaces are often a topic of discussion in relation to injury risks. In Thoroughbred racing, research into racecourse surfaces as a risk factor for injury has a long tradition. In the mid 1980s the famous Newmarket vet Peter Rossdale published a study with a different angle. He looked at injury rates in training among horses with six different trainers. The study showed that the injury risk varied greatly among the six. This helped inspire a new focus on the role of training factors as an injury risk and, in a next step, how best to prevent injury. This has long been a subject of study in human sports injury research. Studies have since shown that training strategies vary between racehorse trainers, with associated differences in injury rates.

BACKGROUND – WHY THIS BOOK?

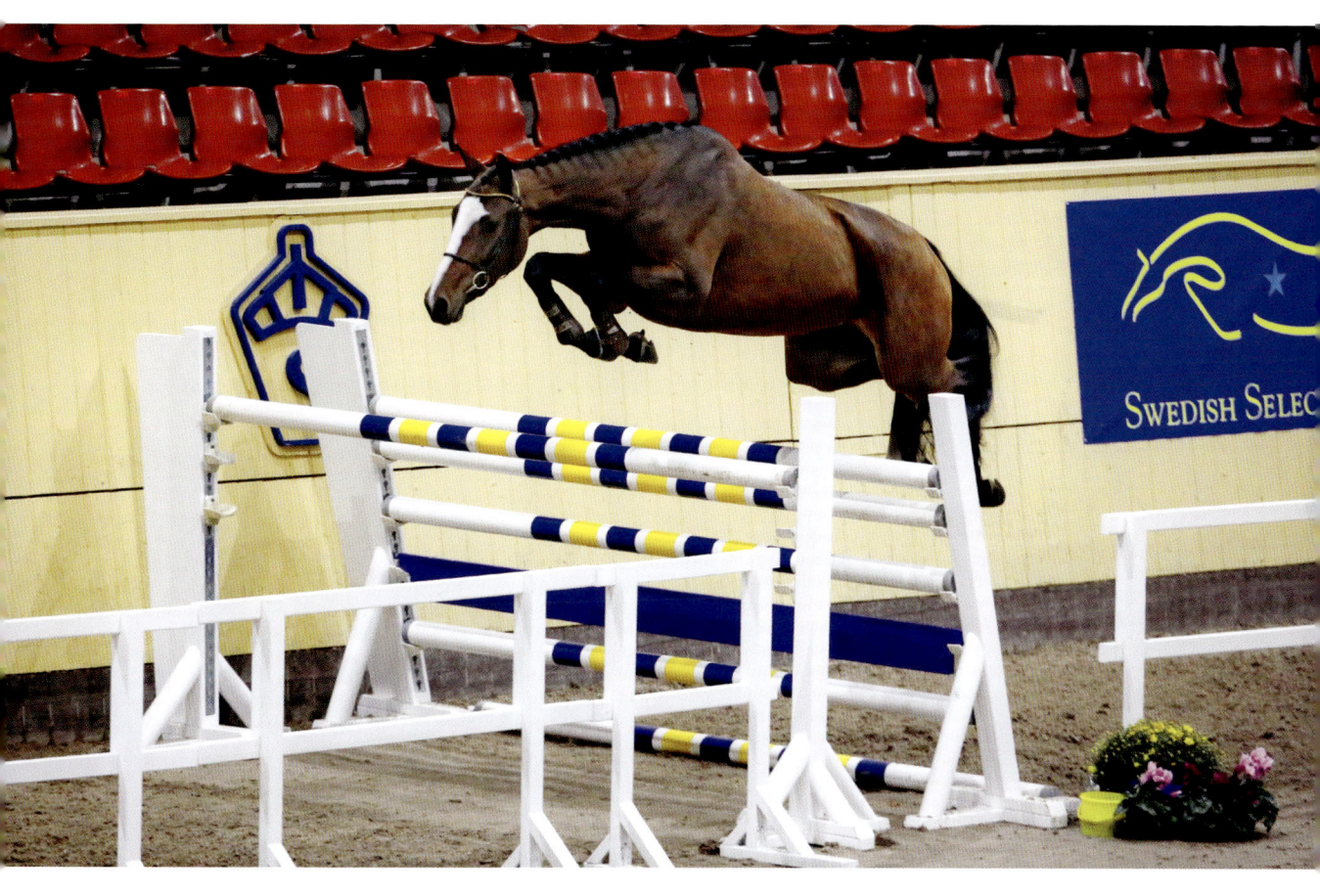

Modern sport horse breeding produces horses with great scope and talent, but training is necessary to help the body prepare for performance demands. *(Photo: Roland Thunholm.)*

Studies of fractures and joint injury in racehorses have underlined a factor that is true also for sport horses (and human athletes); that an orthopaedic injury seldom develops from one day to another, even if the rider or trainer does not observe the first subtle signs. So what is called 'acute' has, in fact, in many cases taken days, weeks or even months, coming. One exception, when injuries can really be called 'acute' is, of course, accidents such as a kick or a fall.

One aspect of equine orthopaedic injury is that the sport horse of today is almost too physically talented for his own good. Modern sport horse breeding has developed horses with a natural, inborn ability to jump big fences or to trot with spectacular action. Riders can then become easily tempted to demand too much performance too soon, especially from a young horse. The young sport horses of today have the genetic potential to perform at a high level, but if the body is not allowed a build-up period, to adapt to the physical demands in training and competition, the risk of injury will be imminent.

You can compare a talented young horse with buying a computer with a great number of gigabytes. The horse also has a high built-in capacity, but before the body is ready for specific training or competition it first needs various 'programmes' installed. Such updates take no more than a few hours in a computer, but months and years in the body of a horse. If you then decide to change what is expected of the horse, including at what level, the 'programmes' need updating, to adjust to the new use. In other words the horse's body needs a re-installation period. Chapter 2, about the horse's body, describes how, while fitness training can quickly give the horse increased heart-lung capacity, the musculoskeletal system with bone, tendons, ligaments and joints, needs longer in order to adapt to increased work demands. This process needs to be done step by step. To repeat; ignoring or minimising that can increase injury risk. It is the same for an athlete or recreational runner. A person can be born with great talent for handling a ball or running, but were he expected to play several matches in a row, or run a marathon without the prior preparation of a conditioning period, injury would be very likely.

It can be easy or tempting to think that riders competing at higher levels than you do it mainly thanks to having better finances and more expensive horses. Of course, there are riders at all levels of competition who are able to afford to improve their chances of rosettes by buying talented horses, getting help in the daily training and paying to be coached by the best trainers, but this does not necessarily translate into long-term success. The highest-ranked riders in the world have, in most cases, got to the very top by being much better than the average rider at making the best out of the horses they have. As former World Champion Jos Lansink says later on in the book, horses are not born as Olympic or World medallists, but are brought on to that level by a skilled rider. In Chapter 4 on finding the right horse there are several examples of champion horses who came with obvious talent but also needed expert handling to realise that talent. You need to work on both your own and the horse's weaknesses, former World Champion Franke Sloothaak has said, commenting: 'It is important that you as a rider understand the horse, what his weaknesses are, which of those you can live with, and which you have to work on. The ability to analyse the individual horse and distinguish his needs is probably the most important challenge for all riders, but also what makes the sport so fascinating.'

Former World Cup Champion and World Number One Daniel Deusser was working for Franke when he first rode professionally. Later, he was one of several champions getting help from the veteran German master trainer Manfred Kötter. Kötter has not sought the limelight but he also coached, for example, the Ludger Beerbaum stable.

'As a rider you might want to get training results in two to three weeks, but Manfred has made me realise that the horse might need two to three months in order to, for example, develop his muscles or change his mental responses', Daniel said in an interview. It was Manfred Kötter who helped Deusser to develop the mare Evita from an ex-broodmare who was jumping 1.40m classes to winning the Rolex Top Ten Final against the other highest-ranked showjumpers in the world in 2013. 'Evita is a special horse, with a lot of scope. She is a big horse with a good character, but she needed work on her body, and time for that', Daniel said. Deusser's analysis of Evita is an example of the fact that, while a horse might have fantastic scope, nevertheless there may be some weakness that needs working on if the inborn talent is to be fulfilled. This skill and intuition is what puts the best riders apart from

'As a rider it can be easy or tempting to think that riders competing at higher levels than yourself do it mainly thanks to having more expensive horses. But the highest-ranked riders in the world in most cases got to the very top by being much better than the average rider at making the best out of the horses they have.'

the rest. Daniel Deusser says that Manfred Kötter has also helped him to develop his patience: 'He has taught me not to focus just on what is a problem with the horse, but on what has actually improved.'

Deusser points out how Evita needed to develop physically. In other sports you talk about physical training versus technical training, and then include exercises and programmes aimed at strengthening the body and helping to prevent injury. The tennis player preparing for matches will not just be hitting balls; the competitive skier does not just train on the slope or on the cross-country ski track. This is important also for horses, and is part of the training strategies used by John Whitaker and other legendary riders. For riders who want to improve their technical skills there are a large number of books and DVDs by top riders and trainers to choose from. You can also attend clinics with top riders and coaches, and get their advice in equestrian magazines and on equestrian TV channels. But, unlike other sports, there is a lot less information available about the physical training of sport horses, about management factors affecting performance and how to prevent injury. Research into training and injury prevention again has a long tradition in Thoroughbred racing, but less so in other equestrian sport.

Inspiration from racehorse research projects contributed to an initiative by the author to study training, arena surfaces and injury in riding horses, starting with riding school horses, in collaboration with more senior colleagues at the Swedish University of Agricultural Sciences at Uppsala. This, in turn, led on to The European Footing and Training Study, with other equine research vets in the UK, Switzerland and the Netherlands, financed by the International Equestrian Federation and World Horse Welfare (see page 52). This project also found that the risk of injury can differ between riders/yards, and with different training/management strategies.

If you compare on the one hand findings from injury research in racehorses and human sports science, results from the few injury and training studies done on riding horses, and on the other hand the experience of international champions and other top riders and equine vets quoted in this book, the conclusions are very similar. Look especially at the bullet point advice on soundness in Chapter 3, with ten champion riders and top sport horse vets. If you take out their names and remove the words 'jumps' and 'dressage movements', the key advice is so similar that it would be difficult to pick out who is who; a champion showjumper, dressage rider, eventing coach or top equine vet? Their conclusions on how to prevent injury and keep the horse confident and motivated are very much alike.

Two of the living legends quoted in this book are the former World Champion Franke Sloothaak and former Olympic, European and World Cup Champion Ludger Beerbaum. They both point out that the rider must think of the horse as a four-legged athlete and that the rider is his manager. To meet up with a trainer once a week is not what, on its own, produces results in the arena or in the long term. It will help, but the deciding factor is rather what double Olympic Gold medallist Beezie Madden describes; the importance of doing what is right in every little detail, day by day. That gives a overview perspective of the management of your horse. Champion riders vary in their systems, but what they have in common is that they all have a system and a plan.

My ambition is to pass on the advice from some of the most successful and most respected veteran riders and well-known equine vets in the world on soundness, training and optimum performance, and show how their thoughts match research findings and fundamental principles of training physiology. This includes having a look at the day-to-day management in top yards and realising that there is plenty to be inspired by.

Sources

The book is based on several independent sources. One is findings from published equine veterinary research, including the author's own equine Ph.D studies, combined with notes from veterinary/equine congress lectures. Another main source is interviews and training features by the author with champion riders and other specialists. Some recent interviews were made specifically for this book, including on soundness advice with Carl Hester at the Dressage Convention at Bury Farm in October 2015 and with John Whitaker at a national show at Aintree the same week. Most articles quoted have been published in *Ridsport*, and the remaining individual ones in *Hippson*, *Showjumping* (last issue in 2015), *Kentaur* and *Häst och Ryttare*, which is the member's magazine of the Swedish Equestrian Federation. In the Swedish version of this book it was stated which interview was published in which magazine, but as the texts are not available in English and in most cases not on line, such detail is not provided here. The two exceptions where other writers are quoted are a review of a clinic with Kyra Kyrklund by Pernilla Linder-Velander in *Ridsport* (on trying out a new horse) and a book and series on conditioning with Charlie Lindberg and Dr Staffan Lidbeck by Ingrid Andersson. Quotes from Michel Robert are mainly from an in-depth interview for *Ridsport*, but also from his excellent book *Secrets of a Great Champion*. Main scientific references with their authors are listed at the end of this book. Some references are given as background to illustrate research in the field, others directly quoted in the text. To the best of my ability I have double-checked all quotes; riders, vets and from scientific articles. My apologies for any mistakes that are present in spite of those efforts.

The author's M. Phil and Ph.D and theses:

M. Phil; Royal Veterinary College, London 2003: 'The use of serum markers of cone cell activity to monitor training and predict injury in the Thoroughbred: A field study'.
Ph.D; Swedish University of Agricultural Sciences 2012: 'Yard differences in training management and orthopaedic injury in Showjumping, riding school and Thoroughbred racehorses'.

BACKGROUND – WHY THIS BOOK?

CVs of quoted champion riders
(alphabetical order)

Showjumping

Ludger Beerbaum, Germany, former World Number One, European individual Champion 1997 (Ratina Z) and 2001 (Gladdys S) (plus 4 x European team gold), Olympic individual Champion 1992 (Classic Touch) plus (3 x team gold medals in 1988,1996 and 2000), World Cup Champion 1993 (Ratina Z), World Championship team gold in 1994 and 1998 plus more than a dozen silver and bronze medals, including team bronze at the 2016 Rio Olympics (Casello). Coached Henrik von Eckermann, Marco Kutscher and Christian Ahlmann to top level.

Rolf Göran Bengtsson, Sweden, former World Number One, Global Champions Tour Champion in 2016 (Casall ASK), European Champion 2011 (Ninja La Silla), won European bronze and silver 2001 (Pialotta), Olympic team silver 2004 (MacKinley), individual Olympic silver 2008 (Ninja La Silla) plus European team bronze 2013, World Championship fourth 2014 (Casall ASK).

Peder Fredricson, Sweden, Junior European Eventing Champion 1989 (Hilly Trip), individual showjumping Olympic silver medallist 2016 (H&M All In), team Olympic silver medallist 2004 (H&M Magic Bengtsson). Also Olympic eventer in 1992.

Jos Lansink, Holland and Belgium, World Champion 2006 (Cumano), World Cup Champion 1994 (Libero H), Olympic team gold 1992 (Egano), plus silver and bronze medals. Now also a coach; former stable jockey Frank Schuttert has reached the Dutch national team.

Beezie Madden, USA, World Cup Champion 2013 (Simon), double team Olympic gold medallist 2004 and 2008 (Authentic), double World Championship silver 2006 (Authentic) and double bronze 2014 (Cortes C), Olympic team silver 2016 (Cortes C). First female rider to reach World Top Ten ranking.

Rodrigo Pessoa, Brazil, Former World Number One, World Champion 1998 (Lianos), Olympic Champion 2004 and World Cup Champion 1998–2001 (Baloubet du Rouet), double Olympic team medallist.

27

SPORT HORSE

Michel Robert, France, Team World Champion 1982 (Ideal de la Hague) and double silver medallist at the 1994 World Championships (Sissi de la Lande), Global Champions Tour Champion in 2009 (Pepita de Kellemoi), plus ten other championship medals. Won his first international Grand Prix in 1971 and in 1972 was Olympic eventer, but switched to only showjumping. Top coach who spotted and helped develop the talent of 2016 Olympic team gold medallist Penelope Lepreveost.

Franke Sloothaak, Germany, World Champion 1994 (Wejhaiwej), Olympic team champion 1988 and 1992 and double team World Champion. Mentor of World Cup Champion Daniel Deusser.

John Whitaker, Great Britain, former World Number One, European Champion 1989 (Milton), double World Cup Champion 1989–1990 (Milton), plus more than twenty additional international championship medals. Head of the phenomenal showjumping family that, in 2015, had ten members in the FEI World rankings.

Peter Wylde, USA, Team Olympic Champion in 2004, World Championship individual bronze medallist 2002 (Fein Cera). Wylde discovered and brought on Hello Sanctos, who in 2014 was the World's highest-ranked showjumper with Scott Brash.

Plus quotes from Malin Baryard-Johnsson, Jens Fredricson and Lisen Bratt-Fredricson, Sweden; Otto Becker and Daniel Deusser, Germany; Henk Nooren, Netherlands; Steve Guerdat and Beat Mändli, Switzerland; Nelson Pessoa, Brazil; Michael Whitaker, UK; Laura Kraut, US.

BACKGROUND – WHY THIS BOOK?

Dressage

Jan Brink, Sweden, Aachen Dressage Champion in 2005 with Briar, seven international championship medals and seven times Swedish Champion. Top dressage coach including of Sweden's 2015 European Young Rider bronze medallist team and the U25 bronze medallist team of 2016.

Carl Hester, UK, Olympic and European Team Champion in 2012 and 2011 (Uthopia), and a further eight international Championship medals since 2009, including team silver at 2016 Olympics (Nip Tuck). Discovered and trained Charlotte Dujardin and the now-retired Olympic Champion Valegro.

Plus quotes from Patrik Kittel and Eric Lette, Sweden; Kyra Kyrklund, Finland; Karin Rehbein and Isabell Werth, Germany; Anky van Grunsven, The Netherlands.

Eventing

Göran 'Yogi' Breisner, Sweden, European Team Champion 1983 (Ultimus). Former assistant of legendary Swedish coach Lars Sederholm. In 1999–2016 UK Performance Manager in eventing (winning five European team golds and four consecutive Olympic medals). In 2017 appointed Olympic High Performance Manager by the Swedish Olympic Committee to work with eventing, dressage and showjumping.

Pippa Funnell, UK, European Champion in 2001 (Supreme Rock) and 2003 (Walk on Star), plus half dozen further medals including 2004 Olympic bronze (Primmore's Pride). Only eventing rider to win the Rolex Grand Slam with successive victories at Badminton, Burghley and Lexington. Also Grand Prix level showjumper and successful coach.

Plus quotes from Karen Donckers, Belgium.

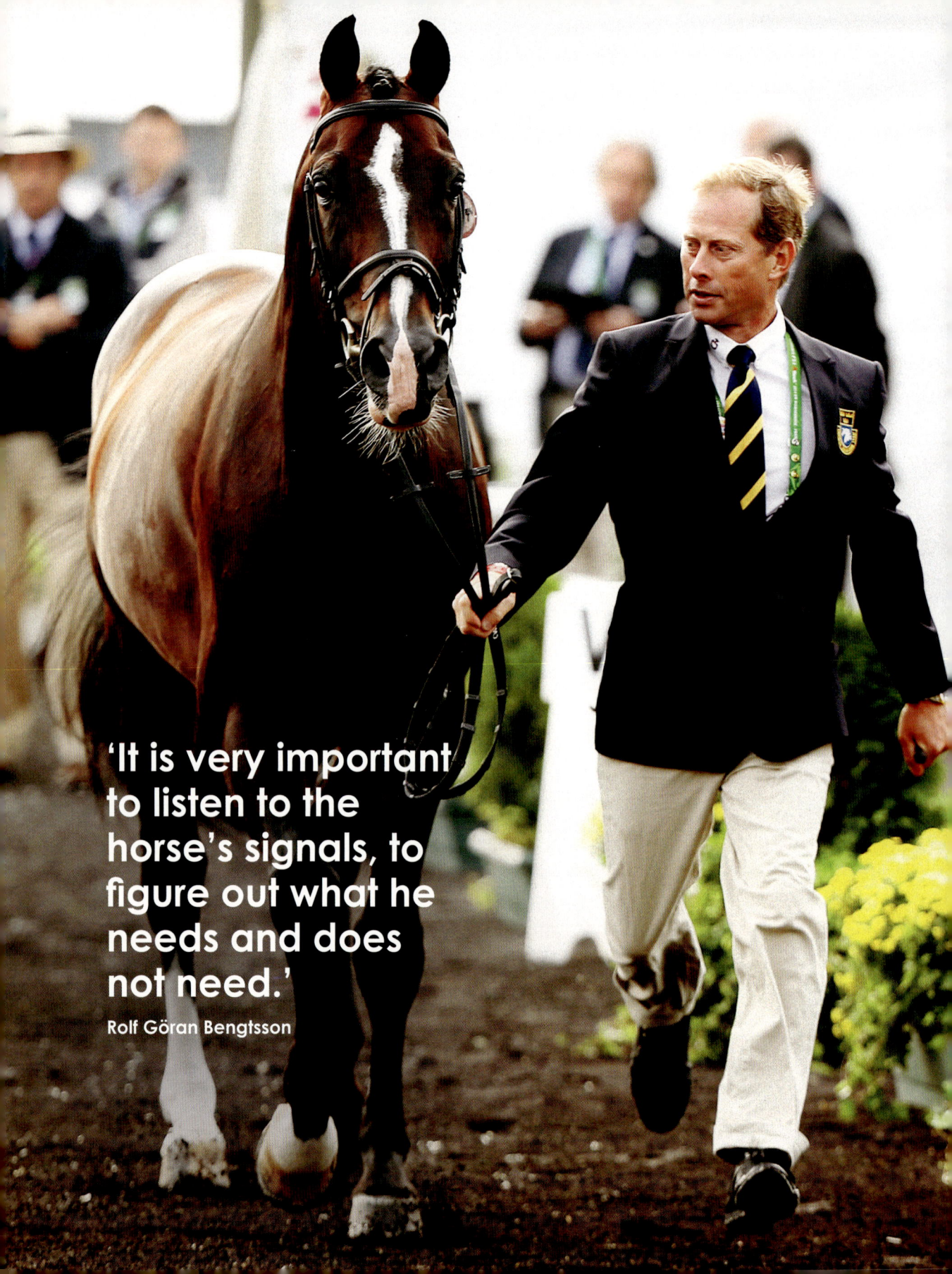

'It is very important to listen to the horse's signals, to figure out what he needs and does not need.'

Rolf Göran Bengtsson

BACKGROUND – WHY THIS BOOK?

CVs quoted equine vets

Dr Hilary Clayton, USA, UK-born vet and scientist, author of one of the few books written on physical training of sport horses. From 1997 to 2014 held the Mary Anne McPhail Dressage Chair in Equine Sports Medicine at Michigan State University. Currently working as President of Sport Horse Science. Has competed in several equestrian disciplines including up to Grand Prix dressage.

Dr Sue Dyson, UK, one of the world's most experienced sport horse vets and researchers, active for over thirty-five years at the equine clinic at the Animal Health Trust in Newmarket. Former event rider herself who, in 2016, was inducted into the University of Kentucky Equine Research Hall of Fame.

Professor Gerhard Forsell, Sweden (1882–1964), Swedish team vet at 1912 Olympics, pioneering surgeon who published some 100 scientific papers. President of the Swedish Veterinary Association 1932–37. Dean of the Swedish Royal Veterinary College 1937–47.

Dr Charlie Lindberg, Sweden, equine vet with some forty years experience, including long-term consultant at the equine insurance department at Agria. FEI vet and horse breeder.

Dr Jonas Tornell, Sweden, equine orthopaedics vet with over thirty years experience and a private clinic – also works with top Standardbred trotters. Swedish team vet in showjumping from 1997 until 2016. Accompanied the team to four Olympics and has been looking after team horses Butterfly Flip, Casall ASK and Briar during their long careers in showjumping and dressage.

Quotes also from **Dr Philippe Benoit, France; Professors Ingvar Fredricson and Lars Roepstorff, Dr Staffan Lidbeck, Dr Sara Nyman, Sweden; Dr Rachel Murray, Professors Renate Weller and Alan Wilson, UK.**

CV other

Xenophon, circa 430–355 bc. Greek cavalry officer and historian who wrote the first known riding handbook.

Opposite: The Holsteiner stallion Casall ASK and Rolf Göran Bengtsson. Casall retired from international competition at 18 years of age in May 2017, 12 years after he first started competing internationally. His home show at Klein Flotbek in Hamburg was chosen as his final appreareance. He and Rolf Göran won the Global Champions Tour Grand Prix. In November 2016 they had won the Global Champions Tour final and series, when Casall was 17 years of age. *(Photo: Roland Thunholm.)*

2. The Horse's Body
– anatomy and function

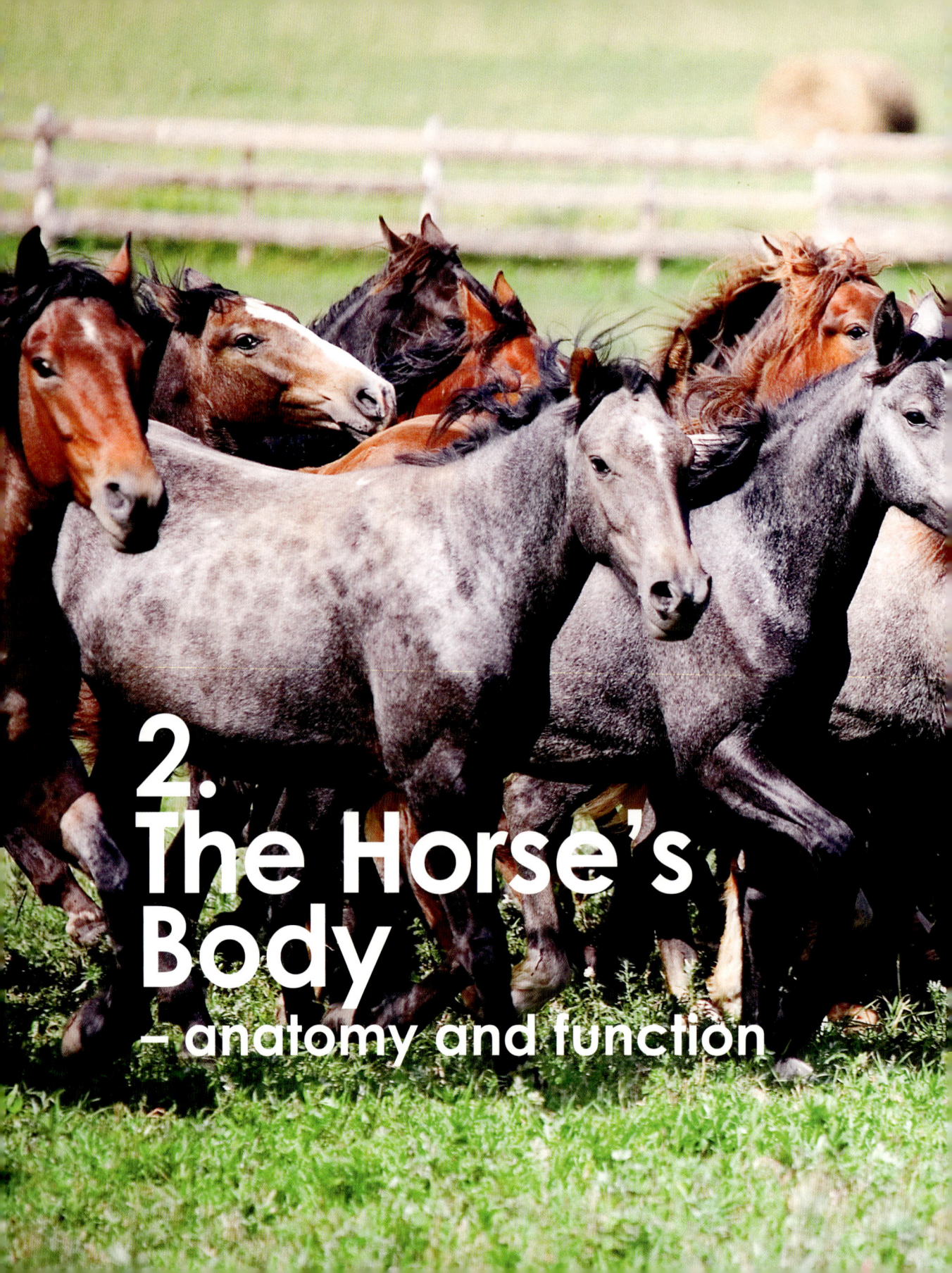

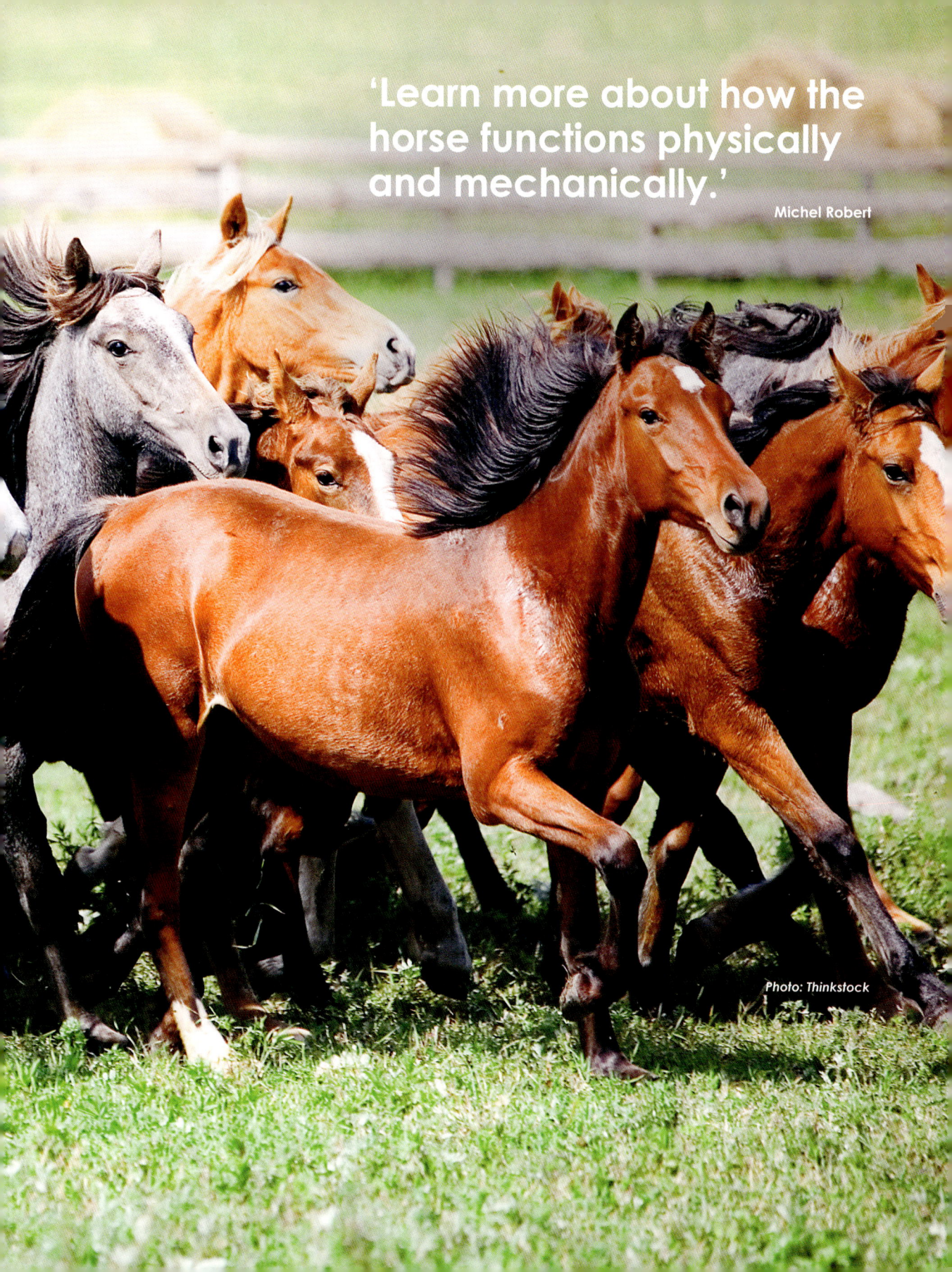

'Learn more about how the horse functions physically and mechanically.'

Michel Robert

Photo: Thinkstock

If you invest time in learning about horse anatomy and how the horse's body functions this can aid both the training process and with keeping the horse sound and healthy.

This will, in turn, strengthen your chances of succeeding as a rider in the long term. Such background is essential in order to understand training at its core; what is reasonable to expect of the horse or not, and how and why injuries happen. Such in-depth know-how of course requires many years of study of books that go into greater detail than this one, plus experience. This chapter is a brief summary. The end of the chapter provides suggestions for further reading and more in-depth detail.

Michel Robert's US colleague Peter Wylde has told how, as a junior rider, he took dressage lessons from a Grand Prix rider. He started reflecting on how the equine body functions, how it is constructed, and how his own body and hands in turn influenced the horse. These insights he has then used in his riding and training.

THE INTERNAL ORGANS

Heart, lungs, spleen, liver and kidneys

While the horse's stomach is small in relation to his body size, the equine heart is large. The heart is a muscle that pumps blood around the body. The blood carries oxygen from the lungs and energy derived from food from the intestines to muscles and all other organs and tissues, and then brings waste products back to the liver and kidneys, to leave the body with the urine and faeces.

When we talk about equine fitness, one key factor is the body's and heart's capacity to transport blood, distributing oxygen and energy. A horse at 450kg has about 34 litres of blood. The heartbeat or pulse is from 20 up to 240 beats per minute (resting rate normally 28–45). The heart of a really fit

THE HORSE'S BODY – ANATOMY AND FUNCTION

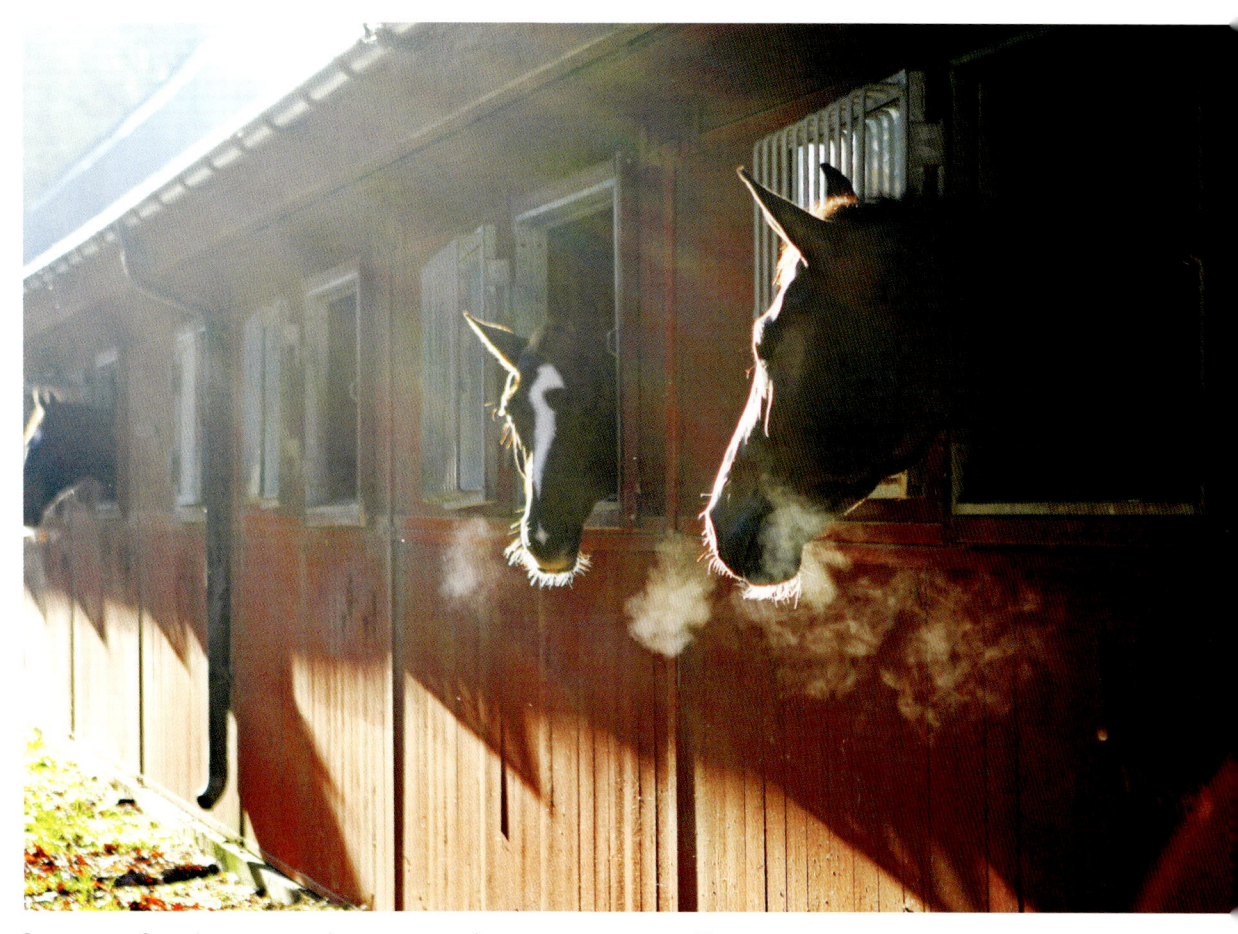

horse performing at maximum capacity can pump 300 litres of blood per minute! But this is above what is required in equestrian sport.

The horse's spleen is a big 'blood bank', releasing extra blood, for example, at times of high exertion. It will then act almost like 'blood doping' in that the horse suddenly has access to more oxygen-carrying red blood cells. An important test of fitness is that the heart rate decreases quickly after training. A high heart rate can be a result of strenuous work, but under other circumstances also indicate pain and illness, for example colic.

Fresh air is a very important prerequisite for a horse to be able to perform. Many top competition stables have specially designed windows that can be opened for the horses to follow what is going on outside. (*Photo: Roland Thunholm.*)

'Blood' horses and big hearts

One traditional expression that has been proven to be true is that some breeds 'have a lot of blood'. It can refer to a horse with lots of energy and nerve, but lighter horses such as Throughbreds or TB-type Warmbloods also have higher volume of blood and greater oxygen carrying capacity in relation to bodyweight than heavier, draught-type breeds. 'A big heart' is another expression, which can refer to a fighting spirit and will to win, but also can be literal. The US popular equine science magazine *The Horse* has offered one rule of thumb that says the horse's heart weighs one per cent of his bodyweight. This would mean 5kg in a 500kg horse, or the size of a large melon. The legendary US racehorse Secretariat had a heart weighing 10kg. That is more than the allowed carry-on luggage weight on many airlines.

Stomach and intestines

The horse has a small stomach in relation to his body size, only eight to 15 litres capacity. The horse is, by nature, a grazing animal, designed for roaming large grasslands or steppes, eating a little at a time but for many hours of the day. His gastrointestinal system is therefore designed to handle grass and its fibre. This is why one important rule in horse care and management is feeding several times a day. Together with orthopaedic injury, gastrointestinal problems, including colic, are one of the most common and serious problems in horses. 'Colic' basically means stomach or gut pain, and can be caused by various problems including impactions, and in serious cases, can result in a twisted gut.

As the horse is, by nature, a grazing animal the modern recommendation is primarily to feed hay or haylage, and of excellent quality. Equine feed scientists including vets specialised in feeding have shown that, with a good-quality hay or haylage, many categories of adult horses do not even need a hard feed with, for example, oats, barley, or corn. As with humans and dogs or cats in affluent countries today, more horses are overfed than underfed. Traditional, starch-rich hard feed has been linked to increased risk of both colic and stomach ulcers. Stomach ulcers is a proven risk for sport and racehorses, and will affect performance negatively. The risk of ulcers is influenced both by feeding and other management factors.

THE MUSCULOSKELETAL SYSTEM

Muscles

Early on in this book are quotes from Ludger Beerbaum and other champion riders who point out that the sport/competition horse is, and needs to be, treated as a four-legged athlete.

An obvious truth for anyone who has been involved in any kind of training is that a muscle will change in response to training (or lack thereof of). The human weightlifter has bigger muscles than the 'couch potato'. But training does not only affect muscle dimensions, but also how effectively they process oxygen and energy. That is a determining factor for the horse's strength and endurance. Think of a showjumper who tires at the end of a jump-off, or a dressage horse who is a bit 'off' in the final class of a competition weekend. Another factor relating to muscles is that different breeds have different muscle-fibre profiles. One type of muscle fibre is used for fast, intensive work, others for slower work that demands more endurance. A Thoroughbred racehorse will have more of the 'fast' fibres; an Arab endurance horse more of the 'slower' kind. While different breeds have different muscle profiles, the fibre composition of an individual will also adjust with training.

One prime factor in determining performance is how effective muscles are at getting oxygen from the blood. If the rate of oxygen delivery matches the rate of exertion, this is known as 'aerobic respiration'. If the rate of exertion is higher than the rate of oxygen delivery, the result is 'anaerobic respiration' at which point the body will start producing lactic acid. With lactic acid the body will tire quickly, but have a very efficient energy source for that short time. If we look at the three Olympic equestrian disciplines we will find that:

1. Dressage work is primarily aerobic (that is, the horse produces little or no lactic acid).
2. Showjumping is primarily aerobic work, but can cause lactic acid production, for example in courses with higher fences and when jumping at higher speeds.
3. Eventing cross-country demands a higher level of exertion from the horse and can give very high lactic acid values.

The horse's legs

We have observed that the horse has a big heart and small stomach in relation to his body size.

What about the legs? They are thin in relation to the rest of the body. Compare the circumference of a horse's leg, that helps carry 450–700kg, with the dimensions of your own legs and what weight they carry!

A narrower, lighter leg can move more quickly, which is a bonus for a prey animal like the horse, or a dressage horse showing light, expressive movement. But if the horse has thin legs in relation to his bodyweight this will also mean that the load per area increases – and probably also the injury risk. This is why some stud books have requirements for minimum cannon bone circumference in stallions. Indeed, around 2,400 years ago Xenophon stated that a good cannon bone was a good indicator of soundness.

Two well-known equine biomechanical experts in the UK are Professors Alan Wilson and Renate Weller at the Royal Veterinary College in London. They have pointed out that, when the horse moves at some speed, the load on a horse's leg is higher than bodyweight alone, and is related to the speed of the horse. Those interested in physics know that this relates to the law that a certain speed times a certain mass (such as the horse's bodyweight) turns into a certain force, that is, load on the leg. In other words this means that the faster you ride the more the load on the leg increases. To give examples:

Walk: half the bodyweight (300kg for a 600kg horse).

Trot: equal to the bodyweight (600kg for a 600kg horse).

Canter: up to 2.5 times the bodyweight (up to 1.5 metric tonnes for a 600kg horse).

This is also something to take into account when looking at the horse's feeding. At the ISES Congress in 2010, UK sport horse vet Sue Dyson listed overfeeding in her warnings relating to unsoundness. If a horse carries 100kg overweight, each leg will be subject to up to 250kg unnecessary load on every leg at each step (based on the principles above)!

The horse's leg as landing gear

Olympic and European medallists Peder and Jens Fredricson's father Professor Ingvar Fredricson was head of Flyinge National Stud during much of their youth, but before that was a pioneer of equine biomechanics by studying horse movement and track surfaces. With the help of engineers at the Saab aerospace division in Linköping, who designed the fighter plane Viggen, he did high-speed filming of Standardbred trotting horses to analyse the pattern of movement and how the hoof makes contact with the ground, in order to make trotting tracks more horse-friendly. If you think of it, the hoof and leg of the horse have a similar job to the landing gear of an aeroplane. When the flight engineers saw the high-speed movies of trotters at top speed and how the hooves hit the ground, one said that 'if we constructed landing gear the way God designed horse's legs, they would break as soon as the plane landed', as the force when the hoof hits the ground is so huge, Fredricson Sr recalls.

Training and adaptation

One definition of orthopaedic injury is that it is a failure of adaptation to training (work)! It is very important to understand that the horse's bones, joint cartilages, ligaments and tendons respond and adapt to training and work, but that this process takes much longer than for the heart, lungs and muscle. If you forget or ignore that, the risk of injury increases.

This is why it is so important that the horse gets variation, rest and recuperation as part of his training regimen. It is during planned rest that the body gets the time to 'rebuild' as a response to training. 'Rest' should not mean that the horse is standing idle in his stable or in a small paddock, but having an relaxing, easy time.

Talking about training and adaptation, there is an important difference between skeletal bone and muscle versus cartilage, tendons and ligaments. Bone and muscle can mend fully after injury. Joint cartilage, tendons and ligaments have more limited capacity for repair, so once an injury had occurred there is a greater risk of re-injury or reduced function.

Bone

The horse's skeleton might appear as a hardy frame that does not change. In fact, bone responds to training just as other tissues in the body, and adapts to different loads (or lack thereof).

As with muscle there are different kinds of skeletal bones, with different roles. Together with tendons, ligaments and cartilage, long bones (primarily in the legs) act as levers in the movement, and short/small bones act as something like suspension springs in the legs. There are also bones such as in the ribcage and skull designed to protect inner tissues. Bone is also a mineral depot for the rest of the body, and it is in the bone marrow that red blood cells are formed.

In horses, as with humans, the skeleton does not adapt to training all over but (as with muscle) mainly in those locations

THE HORSE'S BODY – ANATOMY AND FUNCTION

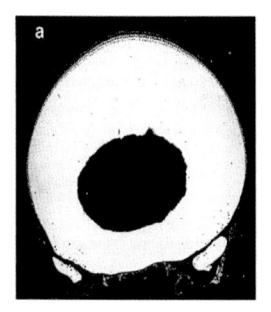

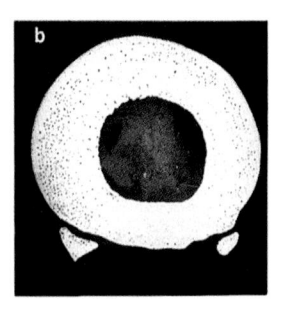

Bone is a hard tissue and it is easy to believe that, unlike for example muscle, it is very constant and does not respond to any training. But the skeleton 'rebuilds' both in response to lack of activity and in response to training. These images show cannon bones in cross-section from a scientific study of equine skeletal response to training. To the left is the cannon bone from a Thoroughbred who was galloping at up to racing speed on a treadmill, and to the right is a 'control' Thoroughbred (for comparison) in the same study, who instead did only walker exercise. Note how the bone of the horse in intense exercise is 'whiter', as a result of adaptation and higher bone density. The bone of the horse who was only on the walker looks 'spotty'; the small black dots reflect lower bone density, because that bone did not have to adapt to galloping. If you compare the two cannon bones they also have different dimensions, also resulting from different adaptation to different loads. As a response to the strain when the galloping leg was hitting the treadmill surface, the front of that leg is 'thicker', compared to the horse who was only on a walker. This is from a racehorse study, but we show the images to demonstrate how differences in adaptation can look. (*Image courtesy of McCarthy and Jeffcott, from* 'Effect of treadmill exercise on cortical bone in the third metacarpal in young horses', *Research in Veterinary Science 1992 52:28–37.*)

Did you know that...

The horse's forelegs do not have any joint connecting them to the rest of the skeleton, as the horse is without collarbones. Instead, the connection of the forelegs to the trunk is through muscles and ligaments. The hind legs, in contrast, have joints to the pelvis. This is one explanation of why the horse can have such a large range of movement in front, upwards over a fence or forward, for example in extensions.

that are loaded. If you check the arms of a right-handed tennis player, the skeletal bone of the right arm will have higher bone density (be stronger) than the left arm, because when hitting the ball the right arm had received signals to adapt that the left arm did not.

Bone has more scope for adaptation in youngsters, and children who are physically active will have a stronger skeleton than those mainly sitting still, a difference that lingers also when they get older. Reflect on that in relation to breeding horses and raising foals!

Joint injury is most common

Analysis of Swedish equine insurance data by Professor Agneta Egenvall and Dr Johanna Penell showed joint injury to be the most common cause of veterinary care claims and horses being put down.

Ligaments and tendons

Bones are held together by ligaments and tendons. One example is the suspensory ligament, which helps support the pastern joint. Another is the superficial digital tendon, which stores energy when the horse moves and helps the leg to 'pop' forward. The superficial digital tendon then acts like a rubber band or a spring, which in turn recoils and stretches. But, as with a rubber band, the risk is that the stretch is too large.

As the leg is quite slender in relation to the horse's bodyweight, the different parts – for example the superficial digital tendon – are also narrow in relation to the load they carry. A tendon is not thicker than a human thumb, and a suspensory ligament even thinner. Unlike rubber bands, it is unusual for these structures to snap, but injuries are common. In addition, tendons and ligaments have a poor blood supply and have limited capacity for healing if injured.

Joints and cartilage

Joint cartilage is, together with skeletal bone, ligament and tendons, an example of supportive tissue. As with bone and muscle, there are different kinds of cartilage. Joint cartilage is called fibrotic; it serves as shock-absorption and provides 'sliding' surfaces. Cartilage has two main ingredients; collagen (as in skin or hair) and proteoglucans. The collagen fibres form a 'net', or framework, on which the other substances are deposited. The turnover for proteoglucans is from thirty days to three years. Proteoglucans can, then, be restored and help to repair an injury, but the turnover of collagen is so slow that it cannot be replaced in the horse's lifetime. Once the collagen framework is damaged it cannot therefore be repaired.

The hoof

The hoof provides the horse's contact with the ground and as has been summarised by Professors Alan Wilson and Renate Weller has three tasks:

THE HORSE'S BODY – ANATOMY AND FUNCTION

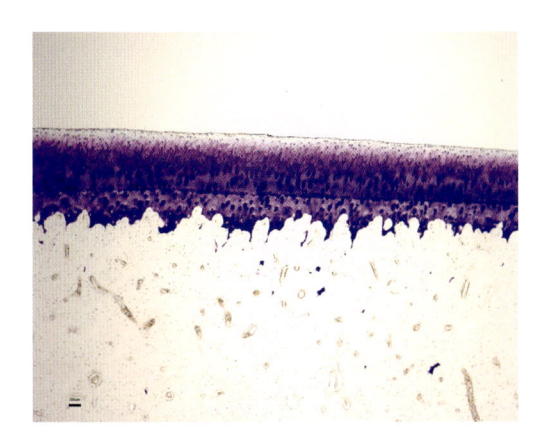

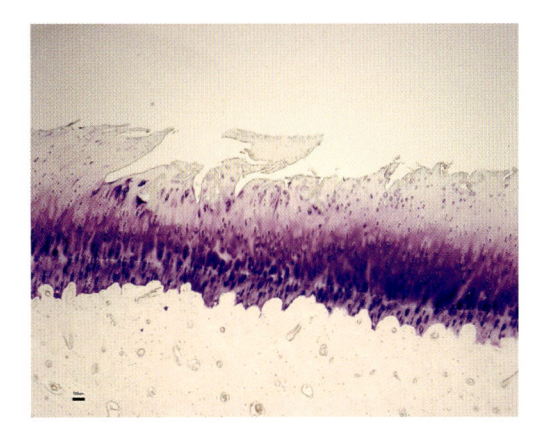

Here we see the difference between healthy and injured joint cartilage in great enlargement. To the left, healthy cartilage, with the smooth surface. To the right, injured joint cartilage, which looks frayed. One challenge in training and competition is to balance demands so that joint cartilage and other tissues are 'primed' for demands in competition, yet are not subject to over- or misuse. Scientific research has shown that physical activity can have an anti-inflammatory effect in the joint and a positive effect on damaged cartilage, but also that an injury process will worsen with continued hard training. (*Images courtesy of Professor Stina Ekman, The Swedish University of Agricultural Sciences.*)

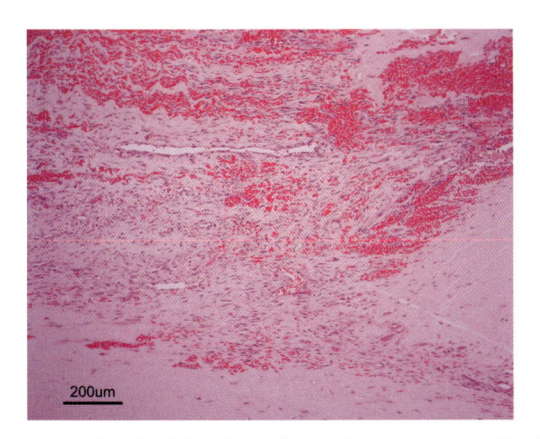

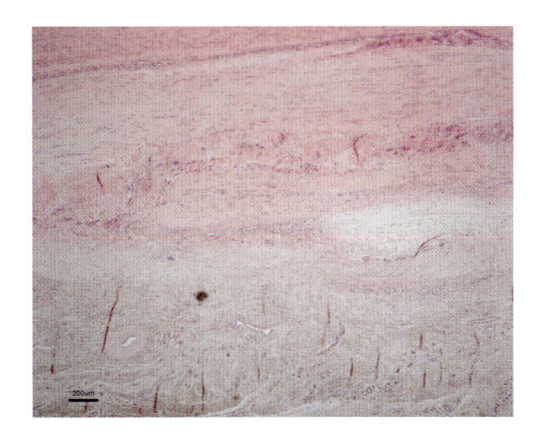

Tendon injury shown in great enlargement; to the right a chronic injury of the superficial digital tendon with scar tissue, to the left a chronic injury that has deteriorated into a rupture with bleeding. What type of training, and the extent to which it can be expected to strengthen a tendon, rather than triggering the start of an injury process that ends like these images, is something that the world's leading experts (in both equine and human tendon research), have not quite agreed on yet. Like cartilage, tendons and ligaments have a narrow interval for what is just right versus too much training. (*Images courtesy of Fredrik Södersten, DVM, The Swedish University of Agricultural Sciences.*)

SPORT HORSE SOUNDNESS AND PERFORMANCE

1. Shock-absorption when the hoof hits the ground.
2. Support and grip when the leg carries the weight of the horse.
3. Traction when the leg leaves the ground.

The angle that the hoof has against the ground in turn affects what effect the hoof impact has higher up in the leg. Compare what a difference it makes for your way of moving if you have different heights and angles on the heels of your shoes. With that in mind it is easy to understand how important correct shoeing and a healthy, strong hoof is for the horse's overall

---

Learn more – reading suggestions

How Your Horse Moves: A Unique Visual Guide to Improving Performance (David and Charles, 2011)
Horse Anatomy for Performance (David and Charles, 2012)
Gillian Higgins and Stephanie Martin

Gillian Higgins has a background in eventing and the ambition to give riders improved understanding and knowledge about the horse's anatomy and biomechanics. She started doing demonstrations painting skeletal bone and muscles on live horses. Such illustrations are used in the books. The first, **How Your Horse Moves** focuses on the locomotion system, especially the skeleton and muscles, and the second, **Anatomy for Performance** describes all body systems.

Activate Your Horse's Core: Unmounted Exercises for Dynamic Mobility, Strength & Balance, Narelle Stubbs and Hilary Clayton (Sport Horse Publications Mason, MI, 2008)

As the title says Hilary Clayton and the Australian equine physiotherapist Narelle Stubbs have also developed exercises on the ground.

Conditioning Sport Horses, Hilary Clayton (Sport Horse Publications, Mason, MI, 1991)

Dr Hilary Clayton's book is one of the few in English on conditioning sport horses written for riders/coaches rather than vets/scientists. Originally written as course material for the Canadian Equestrian Federation's coach training programme. It contains good summaries on equine training physiology, and not only about the Olympic equestrian disciplines of jumping, dressage and eventing but also, for example, endurance and driving.

To really understand more about horse locomotion and training physiology, some other books are also recommended. They are primarily suited for vets and scientists, but can also be read by others with some previous background and interest in anatomy/physiology/biology.

THE HORSE'S BODY – ANATOMY AND FUNCTION

soundness. It is therefore very important to examine the hooves when buying a horse.

The well-known vet and researcher Dr Hilary Clayton gave the same advice as legend Michel Robert early in the chapter: trainers, certainly, but preferably all riders should try to learn how the horse's locomotion system is constructed and works, and about the equine body as a whole. As this chapter is only a short summary, I list here recommendations and suggestions for further reading:

Equine Locomotion, Willem Back and Hilary Clayton (Saunders Elsevier, 2013)

Edited by two of the world's best-known equine biomechanics researchers. Excellent in-depth background. As the title says, the focus is on equine biomechanics, but training physiology is also included.

Biomechanics and physical training of the horse, Jean-Marie Denoix (CRC Press, Taylor and Francis Group, 2014)

Dr Denoix is one of France's (Europe's) best-known sport horse vets and a famous researcher in equine biomechanics. The book does not really discuss training as such, but gives in-depth understanding about how the equine body works in motion, with famous riders and their horses as examples.

Equine Exercise Physiology –The Science of Exercise in the Athletic Horse, Kenneth Hinchcliffe, Raymond Geor, Andris Kanep (Saunders Elsevier, 2008)

This book is a good first choice for understanding more about the horse's body's adaptation to training. As the title says, it covers training physiology as well as some biomechanics. As with Drs Denoix, Back and Clayton for biomechanics, the authors are famous in their field.

For the expert:

The Athletic Horse. Principles and Practice of Equine Sports Medicine, David Hodgson, Kenneth McKeever, Cathy McGowan (Elsevier, 2014)

As with the other titles listed, this book was written by top names in the field of equine exercise physiology and biomechanics. Offers in-depth detailed knowledge and is the most thorough of all, but requires more background knowledge of physiology/biology/medicine. The chapters on actual training are more general, except the one on eventing authored by Olympic gold medallist Wendy Schaeffer.

Photo Bob Langrish

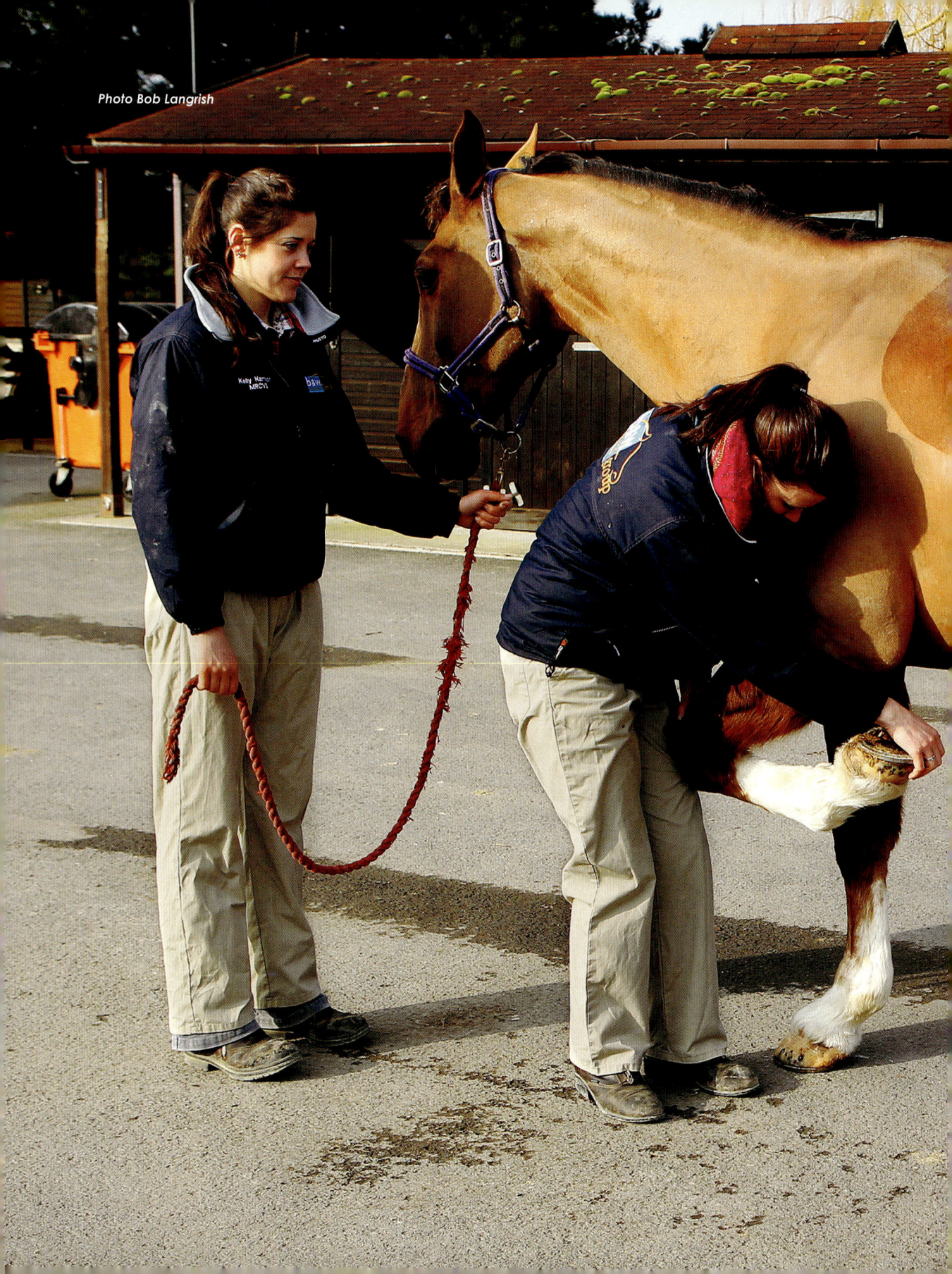

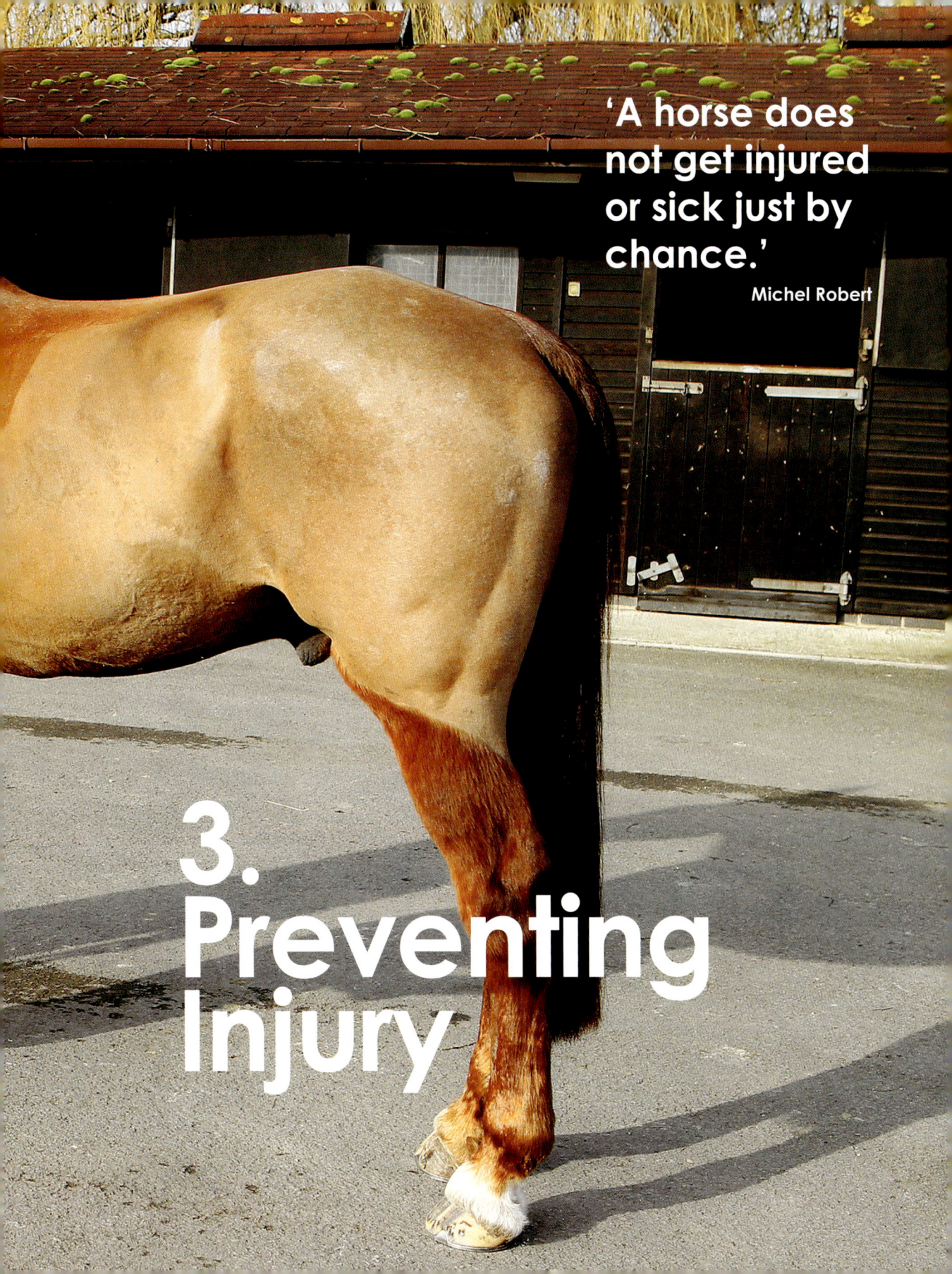

'A horse does not get injured or sick just by chance.'

Michel Robert

3. Preventing Injury

WHAT DOES SCIENTIFIC RESEARCH SAY?

Lameness and other orthopaedic injuries are the major reasons for sport horses to get veterinary treatment. The primary focus is then, of course, to make a diagnosis, treat and rehabilitate. But already by the 1960s Thoroughbred racing had found a different angle; to analyse risk factors for injuries with the aim to prevent them occurring. Prevention of injury based on identification of risk factors is a huge field in human sports science and medicine.

Lamenesses in horses are often described as being caused by 'overuse', or 'wear and tear'. But non-acute injury is more a question of misuse, or inappropriate training and work that has not been adjusted to the individual horse or his level of training and fitness. Orthopaedic injuries are therefore, frequently not just the result of 'bad luck' or chance.

Rather, scientific research points to the fact that sport injuries in both human athletes and horses are often preventable, by appropriate training. Studies aimed at prevention of fractures and other injuries in racehorses first focused on racecourse properties during racing, for example hardness. But, as described in Chapter 9, racehorse studies have also analysed training factors in relation to injuries, and have found associations between different training strategies and risk of, for example, fracture. These research methods have since also been used on showjumping horses, and for arena surface research in studies financed by FEI and World Horse Welfare, among other bodies.

Research findings point to the fact that training-related orthopaedic injuries in both human athletes and horses can be prevented by appropriate training strategies.

No matter how careful and skilled a training and competition programme is, bad luck and individual weaknesses in the horse may still result in an accident or injury. But both experience and science show that, for humans and horses, there are certain situations and conditions when injury is more likely to occur. Have them in mind when planning your training programme or competitions. Here is the list, with examples of how it applies to equine studies.

Different disciplines – different injuries

How different training regimens or work affect injury risk is shown in a case analysis of tendon and ligament injuries from the Animal Health Trust's equine (sport horse) clinic in Newmarket, England. The veterinary researchers, led by Dr Rachel Murray, compared horses from different disciplines who visited the clinic. This showed that some injuries are more common in certain disciplines, and at different levels within that discipline. Examples :

- Horses at advanced level in showjumping and eventing were more at risk of injuries of the superficial digital flexor tendon.
- Jumping horses at advanced level were more at risk of injuries of the deep digital flexor tendon.
- Dressage horses at both higher and lower levels were instead more at risk of injuries of the hind suspensory ligament.

SPORT HORSE SOUNDNESS AND PERFORMANCE

Seven common causes of injury

1. Rapid increase of workload/training.
That is doing too much too quickly. Research aimed at prevention of fracture in racehorses by a UK group led by Professor James Wood and Dr Kristien Verheyen found an increased risk of fracture and joint injury in young Thoroughbreds who had an increase of fast work in a short timeframe, so a rapid increase of workload.

2. Lack of continuity.
A classic problem in human sports medicine, also known as the 'weekend warrior' syndrome. Refers to going to the gym or running but ending up doing only occasional efforts, and often a variation of point 1 – doing too much too quickly.

3. Repetitive training/lack of variation.
One common cause of injury is repetitive work. Think overuse injuries in the workplace. A study of jumping horses trained by elite riders in four European countries (the FEI/WHW training and footing project) found that variation of training was strongly associated with prevention of loss of training days, to the extent that it was 'dose-related' (the more variation, the less risk of days lost to training).

4. Lack of rest and recovery.
One fundamental need for the body when adapting to training and during work periods is planned rest and recovery, The body needs time slots in order to reconstruct or to repair small injuries. One study of riding school horses showed that one management factor in riding schools with the least amount of orthopaedic injury was having a minimum of four weeks summer rest out on grass (24/7 with no riding).

5. Sudden change in workload, or a sudden single overload event.
A variation of point 1, of acute overload. This can be a sudden event such as a wrong step, but there we are back at point 3. The body of a horse who gets varied work on a variety of surfaces will be better prepared for different types of loading.

6. Individual weaknesses including re-injury.

One common risk factor for orthopaedic injury is re-injury. But, in addition, horses (like humans) are more or less hardy, and adapt to training in different ways. We will discuss these individual differences in the next chapter about choosing the right horse. When UK scientists tested the strength of superficial digital tendons in a laboratory setting, some tendons were stronger than others. This means that if two horses do exactly the same work one can get an overuse injury when the other horse stays sound. This is why a key message by several of the champion riders and sport horse vets in this book is the importance of 'listening' to the horse, being observant to his signals and behaviour, and preferably doing daily checks to spot early signs of any injury.

7. Volume and intensity – hard work and lots of work.

One of the biggest challenges in all training is finding the right balance of demands, including volume versus intensity. Depending on your level, the training needs to be demanding enough to prepare for the level of competition, and yet measured to avoid overloading. The higher the level of competition you are at, the tighter that balance will be. One important piece of advice on the prevention of fractures in racehorses can also be applied to conditioning sport horses; when you are at a stage where you increase demands in training, for example by jumping bigger fences or doing faster canter work, you can counteract that by reducing the volume and making the session shorter. Then you can increase the volume again step by step.

The European Footing and Training Study

In 2008 the International Equestrian Federation (FEI) and the UK equine protection charity World Horse Welfare gave scientific funding to a research collaboration between equine vets and researchers in four European countries. The aim was to develop arena surface testing, and analyse associations between training factors, surface use and injury of showjumping horses in professional training. The project was led by Professor Lars Roepstorff and Professor Agneta Egenvall at the Swedish University of Agricultural Sciences at Uppsala, and had two Ph.D students; the author of this book on training and Elin Hernlund on surfaces. All four are vets.

The training study commenced in 2009 with top-level showjumping riders in Sweden, the Netherlands, the UK and Switzerland. In total 31 riders with 263 horses participated. (The choice of studying professional riders was in part precisely because they work with several horses.) It would have been very cumbersome to analyse training of 263 horses with as many different riders).

The riders filled in daily training protocols (in effect training diaries) for up to six months. They registered each horse's daily activity and timeframes: whether he was jumping, or going hacking, or doing flatwork and for how long; at what perceived intensity; and any non-ridden activity such as being in the paddock. They also registered if the horse lost training days owing to being injured or sick, or resting for other reasons. They also noted what type of surface the horse was ridden on during each training session.

Results from the study have been published in two scientific papers included in the author's Ph.D, and are quoted in Chapter 8 about training strategies.

The riding surface part of the project is still ongoing at the time of writing, and the training part has offshoots pending. The surface testing started with the riders' home arenas, but also included competition arenas in Sweden and internationally. Professor Lars Roepstorff and (now Dr) Elin Hernlund were consultants in the design of the arena surface at the 2012 Olympics in London, and Professor Roepstorff was again in that role for Rio 2016.

To read more about the surface study findings and riding surfaces, please see Chapter 8 and read the FEI's 'Equestrian_ Surfaces-A_Guide', which Chapter 8 is largely based on. It is a web-based pdf available on the FEI website.

Eventing

In eventing there have been some studies on risk factors for falls in competition, aimed at the prevention of fatalities to riders that had a peak at the end of the 1990s. One group involved in these studies was led by Dr Ellen Singer in the UK. She reported that 21 per cent of horses aimed at starting at international level (CIC) did not start due to injury. Another UK study showed that 35.1% of event horses were not re-registered for competition the next year because of veterinary problems. Singer noted that there is a lack of studies on risk factors for injury in eventing horses. Event horses do get the variation in training recommended elsewhere, but one challenge is, instead, the balance of intensity and volume. Eventing horses have higher demands of speed and fitness in competition than showjumpers or dressage horses. The higher intensity this requires can be a risk factor in itself.

A study at the veterinary faculty in Utrecht by Caroline Munsters and colleagues showed that Dutch team horses (both ponies and horses) who showed good results in fitness tests early in the season were more likely to start at the European Championships later the same season, and that those with lower fitness were more likely to be out because of injury later on.

Injury patterns

Whether studying jumping yards, riding schools or racing yards, research show differences in the rate of injury between yards. This, in turn, is associated with differences in training strategies and/or horse management.

The scientific field for finding out those kinds of patterns is called epidemiology. One basic assumption in epidemiology is that disease do not occur randomly.

French jumping legend Michel Robert came to the same conclusion after over forty years in international competitions. 'A horse does not become sick or lame by chance', he wrote

What does 'lost training days' mean?

How many days of training or competition did you miss in the past month or year because your horse was sick or injured? In sports and equine injury research this number is called 'days lost to training'. In human sports medicine one use is as a measure of how serious an injury is, but it can also be used to compare rate of injury between yards. Studies of racehorses and showjumpers have shown that injury risk, as measured by percentage of days lost to training, does vary between yards/trainers/riders.

SPORT HORSE SOUNDNESS AND PERFORMANCE

Research into prevention of injury is time-consuming. In 1992 a Dutch scientist named van Mechelen published a golden standard or guideline for research on prevention of human sports injury. The stages are:

1. Study how common a certain injury is.
2. Study possible risk factors.
3. Do a training study where the suspected risk factor/s are modified or eliminated.
4. Return to point 1 to test whether the changes in training led to a reduction of the number of cases!

This has been done for different types of injury in different human sports, and for racehorse fractures. But studies of sport horse injury has only reached phase 2 as yet. To reach phase 4 will take at least another decade. There are, at the same time, biological principles for what benefits the body (or not) in training, and in this book I have elected to combine and discuss scientific results from both human sport injury studies, equine injury studies and experience-based knowledge from veteran riders and vets. One remaining scientific challenge is finding methods to pinpoint the elements of correct versus incorrect riding, that are benefits against what could be damaging to the horse. Technical developments including high speed imaging is enabling biomechanics researchers to develop this field.

in his book *Secrets of a Great Champion*. 'When he does it is rather like a red warning lamp saying "Be careful, you are not training in the right way." Why do horses in one stable tend to have problems with their hocks? And why is it in another yard always the same part of the back that horses have problems with?'

One aim of epidemiological studies is to identify potential risk factors, in order to prevent new cases. One early example of epidemiological research was the discovery that smokers run an increased risk of developing lung cancer.

There is a study of soccer teams at Champions' League level that show that certain coaches bring with them certain player injury patterns when they change clubs. This means that different teams of players get the same type of injury when they have the same coach – so a pattern emerges very much like Michel Robert's comment about yard differences and this, again, fits with results from veterinary research. Unsurprisingly, the pattern of injury in the soccer teams also affected their results in the Champions' League. More injuries

Differences in injury risk between trainers/yards

Another way to measure the risk of injury is cases per horse/month; 100 horses in one yard during one month equals 100 horse/months, or 10 horses for ten months is also 100 horse/ months.

- Fracture-risk racehorses: from zero to 5.26 fractures per 100 horse/months (or a little more than five fractures in one month with 100 horses in the yard).
- Joint injury racehorses: some trainers had 0.4 joint injuries per 100 horse/months (less than one per month with 100 horses in the yard), while others had up to the equivalent of seven cases of joint injury per 100 horse/months.
- Orthopaedic injury riding school horses: there are riding schools that, year after year, have hardly any cases measured as insurance claims, while others have the equivalent of 33 claims per 100 horses in a year.

resulted in poorer results – again an example that soundness and success are associated.

Soundness and know-how

Do know-how and experience help in injury prevention? It would make sense to think so, and later in this chapter both Ludger Beerbaum and Jan Brink mentions learning from mistakes when discussing their bullet point advice on soundness. A UK study of tendon injury in hurdle racehorses showed the risk was lower among horses with more successful trainers. In a study of Swedish riding school horses, based on both insurance claims data and field study visits, a majority of riding schools with a very low rate of injury had managers with long experience. The mean was 18.5 years, compared to a mean of ten years in a group of riding schools with a very high rate of injury claims. In addition, in the group with least injuries, seven out of ten chief riding teachers had a Level 3 (the highest) riding teacher degree, compared to one out of nine in the group with most injuries. Similar observations that riding schools with experienced managers had healthier horses were done in the 1970s, when vet Lars Erik Magnusson visited dozens of Swedish riding schools to review the health status of the horses. The reasons for the differences are difficult to determine scientifically, but comments made by participating riding school representatives indicate one: inexperienced staff and riding teachers/managers are less likely to spot and address early signs of injury, such as staleness, compared to more experienced and better-trained staff. A horse who is recognised as needing a rest might recover without further problems, while a horse kept in work might deteriorate and develop a full-blown injury. This is the same advice as given by Jan Brink for dressage horses.

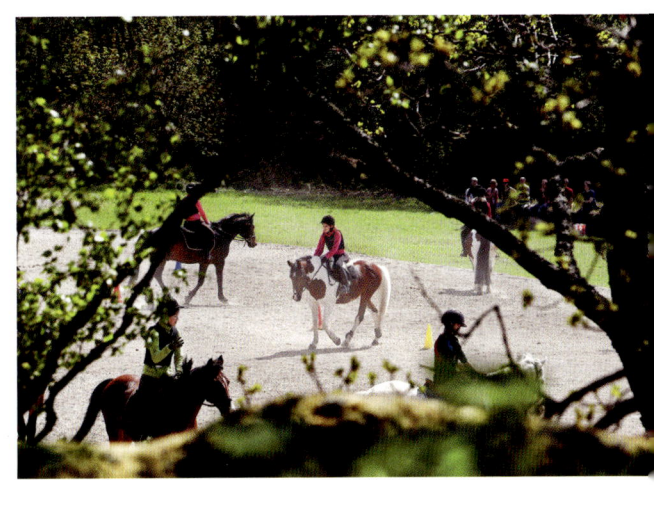

In 1976, that year's Olympic Showjumping Champion Alwin Schockemöhle was asked in an interview about Sweden's chances of becoming a successful showjumping nation. At the time Swedish showjumpers had only occasional international success, and the sport was not big at national level either. Schockemöhle replied that he thought the chances were slim, as riding in Sweden was not a big sport and, without the grassroots, it is more difficult to find and develop top riders. But at the same time in the mid-1970s more and more new riding schools opened, and the Göteborg International Horse Show was started – in effect by a riding school club, Clareberg. Since then several of Sweden's best-known riders have started their careers as riding school pupils, including Malin Baryard-Johnsson, Maria Gretzer and Jan Brink. (*Photo: Roland Thunholm.*)

WHAT DO CHAMPION RIDERS AND TOP VETS SAY?

Research shows that injury can be less down to bad luck and more to training or management factors. The skill necessary to keep the horse sound and healthy is very important for a rider who wishes to stay at top level – or for a rider at any level who wishes to get consistent results. Last, but certainly not least, it is of course also important for the horse's wellbeing. Riders quoted in this chapter are examples of those who have had consistent top-level results over time, and have had horses with long careers in the sport.

When the world's leading riders are asked to share advice it is normally about technical training and skills. Much more seldom are the questions about their huge experience of basic training and about keeping the competition horse confident and motivated.

The idea for this bullet point advice on soundness came from a lecture by the famous sport horse vet Dr Sue Dyson from Newmarket at the ISES Conference at Uppsala in 2010, where she had been asked to talk specifically about soundness factors. One of showjumping's most respected veterans, Beezie Madden, received a similar request on her website from a fan, who noted that her horses tend to last long in the sport, and asked for advice on how she achieves this.

In the preparation for this book the same question was asked to an additional eight of the sport's most veteran and respected names, both champion riders (and one coach) and equine vets. Study them and compare! You will see how strikingly similar they are in their thoughts, irrespective of discipline. Both Ludger Beerbaum and Jan Brink specifically also mention that experience is an important factor when learning to prevent injury. It is that in-depth experience that they and the others are kind enough to share here.

Beezie Madden (jumping)

- Find the right horse for the job. Pay attention to the horse's conformation, and learn to take advice on which problems could be career-ending. Never buy a horse without a thorough vet's inspection.

- The next factor I would mention is to build the horse's fitness in the right way and be selective in the training. Our horses are well prepared to do the job we are asking for, but we achieve this by a varied training regimen, *not* by jumping 1.50m courses every week. At home we seldom jump a whole course of fences at competition height. Instead we often work our horses in gridwork or over fences that are smaller than those we meet in competition. We build the horses' fitness by turnout in the field, on the walker, lots of flatwork and hacking in varied terrain.

- Vary the surfaces you ride on! (Advice from George H. Morris.)

- We ration how much the horses show. When our horses are out competing they seldom do more than two or three classes in a week, and they seldom compete two weeks in a row. At the end of the year they get a complete rest from competition, without shoes and with lots of turnout time in the field over a period of six to eight weeks, so that they get to 'be a horse' and can relax.

- Correct feeding is a cornerstone in our programme.

- Good hay is the basis of our feeding regimen and I am sure we give more hay than most yards in the US, twelve to fourteen 'flakes' [i.e. sections] per day. Almost all hay we give is first crop. We see a lot fewer stable vices when our horses get really good hay. I have no doubt that happy horses perform better. We regularly send in hay samples for nutrition and hygiene analysis, and our grooms are very careful about checking bales and discarding those with any signs of mould or dust. The hard feed we give is trusted high quality feed, which is one of my sponsors. When we first started discussing a contract, my husband John demanded that we could first use the feed for one year as a trial, before we were prepared to sign a contract about promoting it. We have been very impressed by their research and know-how and have learnt a lot from the advice we have received.

- Before you spend a lot of money on supplements it is important first to be sure that you have done everything right for the horse regarding the fundamentals, roughage and hard feed. We give one joint supplement called Hyaloronex, and electrolytes when needed, but these are the only supplements we give.

- Have a good team with equine vets, blacksmith and grooms/staff who are focused on your horses' well-being.

- Put together all the details in the right way and pay daily attention to all the small details.

Own blog January 2014

Carl Hester (dressage)

- To start with it is important that the horse gets to move and be active every day, and not just during the training session.

- The training, how you ride, is important, including varying the training. Do not just do dressage movements the whole time, because you then put wear and tear on the horse. Our horses are only ridden in an arena four days a week. Two days they are hacked out instead, and one day they are just in the field. The fact that they do not only do dressage work is, I think, good for them mentally.

- Fitness work is important. We have hills at home where we work them to develop muscle and the lungs.

- Vary the riding and use different surfaces, so that the horse does not work on the same surface day after day.

- It is important to let the horse warm up and cool down before and after training. Our horses warm up by a 30 minute hack in walk and trot on the roads, and afterwards they get to cool down. When Charlotte and I work the horses it is only for 15–20 minutes.

- Feeding is important. This includes being careful not to overfeed the horse so that he would have to carry surplus weight.

Interview October 2015

John Whitaker (jumping)

- Number one is to see and deal with the horse as an individual, understand and try to figure out what makes this particular horse tick, what he needs. Don't complicate the training but keep it simple. Keep the horse happy and give him a good life, that is as natural as possible.

- Pay attention to the horse's daily 'form'. I want to tack up my horses myself, because I want to keep a check on how they are feeling. I go into his stable, and look to see if he seems as usual, or not. Has he eaten his feed? Does he have clean water? The grooms don't always pay attention to that – well the best ones do, but not all.

- Ration your jumping. Don't compete too much. It is no secret that this makes a difference. Some riders jump and jump and jump, first at home when training and then in the warm-up, and compete often. With my international horses I hardly jump at all at home. If you ration the jumping I think horses last longer, because it gives less wear and tear. Young horses I do a bit more jumping with at home, because they need the education. Then I jump them on Tuesdays, but only ten to twelve jumps. If the horse goes well then that is his only jumping training session that week. If the session does not go so well I will jump him over a few fences the next day as well. Older horses I do not jump at home if they are in a competition period. Horses who have had a break I start off by a few jumping sessions at home before they return to competition.

- I let them go in the field as much as possible. All my horses go out on grass every day. Gammon, who I had in the 1990s, was difficult in the beginning and found it difficult to relax. I started letting him out in the field as soon as we got back from competitions, unless the weather was really bad. Then he was left out in the field for two or three days and overnight. Then he got completely relaxed.

- Varied training. I ride out a lot, on our fields and on the small roads around us, so that the horses do not just have to go around and around in an arena.

- Fitness work. We do roadwork, so walking and trotting on roads and in the fields; we also do hill work and canter work to build their fitness. When my brothers and I grew up we only had the hilly terrain around the farm for riding. We only had a small outdoor arena, and it was on a slope, so we rode in the fields and on the lanes and noticed that it had a good effect.

- I almost forgot; the rider's own balance. It is important for the horse that the rider has his own balance. Some have it naturally, some need to work on it.

Interview October 2015

Jan Brink (dressage)

- To start with it is obviously important what horse you choose. You can have bad luck (look at people, there are clean-living individuals who still get a heart attack). But you can look at the breeding and the other progeny of the sire and dam, and that the conformation is correct.

- One common mistake is doing too much too soon, to make too big demands early on with a young horse. Number one is not to progress too quickly. I think many riders are a bit overambitious and do too much when the horses are young – and this includes experienced, good riders. Then it is easy to spoil the horse and get injuries.

- The volume of training is a factor, especially if you do not give the horse some breaks in the session. Long sessions are not good and you should not have too long, uninterrupted sessions of trot or canter within a session. If you do that the injuries will appear. Make mini-breaks for rest at a walk!

- Vary the training during the week and plan and distribute the work so that, for example, you do not train collected work several days in a row. Go for a ride in the forest in between, vary between collected work and sessions where the horse can be in a bit longer frame, such as changes.

- Vary the types of surfaces you ride on. It is a boon both for the horse's legs and his brain to get outside; walk on tarmac, ride on grass.

- Do not make the same demands in daily training as you would in competition. You do not need to ride half-passes for a mark of '11' every day, and you should ration your extended trots.

- Give the horse time for recovery and rest when he has competed and travelled.

- Let the horse be a horse, be loose out in a paddock and have a roll. Then he will store energy in a good way.

- When you have planned your competitions, make a point of still listening to the horse and skip one or more shows if the horse feels tired and weary. If you push on in spite of the horse not being 100 per cent the big problem injuries occur.

- Let your vet do regular check-ups, so that you catch small problems in time and can give the horse a break. I let Dr Jonas Tornell check on Briar after every fourth show.

- Shoeing is extremely important; pay a lot of attention to that. The mouth is also important, that the horse does not feel uncomfortable in the mouth.

Interview November 2015

Ludger Beerbaum (jumping)

- Number one is to be careful about getting to know the new horse when he arrives, accept his age and learn how weak or strong he is. Then adapt your training to the horse's stage of fitness at this moment. Do not aim for the first competition in, for example, two months time without first analysing and being clear about where the horse stands fitness-wise. That is the quickest way to ruin a horse.

- Pay attention to what the vet inspection showed and discuss it with your vet and blacksmith. It is *very* important that the horse gets good shoeing. Once the horse is in work it is, for example, important that he is not too long in the toe, but get a breakover.

- When you have started working the horse, ask yourself how he feels. Does he seem to find the work easy; is he positive or sour? Does he resist you? Such bodily signals in the daily work are very important to observe and listen to, and then adjust the work accordingly.

- Feeding is also important. That the horse gets plenty – and good – water is important.

- To keep the horse sound and healthy is to a great extent down to experience. You learn from your mistakes.

Interview May 2015

Dr Hilary Clayton (sport horse vet)

- Do not do the same thing every day in training (doing the same thing day after day on the same surface is a common mistake among dressage riders).

- Use nature in your training. Some riders are nervous about going hacking outside. But it becomes a vicious circle, so that if the horse is finally taken on a ride outside he goes wild, so it needs to be done continuously.

- My horses go in a paddock every day as well. One common mistake is to not let a horse be a horse.

- Do not be afraid of including (planned) rest days in the training.

Interview June 2015

Rolf Göran Bengtsson (jumping)

- It is very important to listen to the horse's signals; analyse what he needs and does not need. This is the first point.

- Give the horse time during training and build him up gradually. Some riders expect that everything basically already happened yesterday. But the horse must be allowed time. You only need to look at yourself if you start a fitness programme. You can't do everything in one go, or else you get sore muscles and aches. And if you don't then allow yourself time to recover it only gets worse.

- It is important to set up a sensible competition plan, over time and for the individual show. One example is that you sometimes do not go for victory in the Friday class, if you are doing the Grand Prix on the Sunday. It is a question of management.

- You must pay attention that the horse is ridden and exercised properly and again is allowed to build fitness. At home we are fortunate to have a large arena where we can do canter work, and not just have an indoor of 20 x 60m. We also have a galloping track where we take them out now and then. We do not canter really fast, but at a good speed, and a bit faster sometimes, without making a race out of it.

- It is also important that the horse is ridden in a manner that means he does not accumulate stress and tension, but is relaxed.

- Regular vet checks are important. I first listen to the signals from the horse and describe them to the vet: 'I can feel this or that', and then we analyse it and the vet might say that 'it is nothing to worry about', or that 'this we need to do something about'. That is very important.

- It is also important to have the right equipment with the right fit, so that, for example, there is not a problem with the saddle and the horse gets a sore back from that.

- Ride the horse on different surfaces and not just on one arena, but vary the properties.

Interview June 2015

Dr Jonas Tornell (sport horse vet)

- Get a sound and healthy horse, it is difficult enough anyway (in other words: don't buy problems).

- Pay constant and objective attention to what is reasonable to ask of the horse right now. If, for example, you have a talented young horse who is not quite mature physically, abstain from all young horse championships and work him on a level where injuries are more easily avoided. In that way the horse gets the chance to develop and mature with time.

- The fewer setbacks through injury you have (thanks to avoiding premature high demands), the stronger the horse will become and the greater the chance that his full potential can be realised in the long term.

- Pre-plan the season carefully – ration your competitions and include both training periods, rest and recovery along with shows in the plan.

- Prepare the horse on different surfaces, based on where you will be competing. If the horse will be competing on grass include training on grass; if he will be competing on sand, prepare him on sand.

- Get to know your horse really well and pay attention to any variations in how he feels on a daily basis. Only when you know your horse well will you be able to judge when you can train and when the horse instead needs to have easier work or a break.

- Develop a good co-operation with a small team of experts; an equine vet, a blacksmith and the groom/stable staff, so that you all know your own role and not too many outsiders get involved. All top riders and top trainers who I work with co-operate with and trust their team, and let the vet be the vet. The vet in his/her turn should discuss the horse with the rider or trainer in their vocabulary, not with specialist words as with another vet.

- Always strive to learn more about training, feeding, technical skills, etc., but make sure to have a solid knowledge base and don't divert from it just because some outsider likes to offer opinions.

Interview September 2015

Dr Sue Dyson (sport horse vet)

- Avoid horses with potential problems such as poor breeding, lack of natural balance or poor conformation (for example, different-sized front hooves, straight hocks, straight pasterns).

- Careful trimming and shoeing is important.

- Pay attention to giving the horse sufficient time for warming up and cooling down before and after every training session.

- Increase training gradually and consistently.

- Vary the training (i.e. cross-training).

- Include fitness work to give the horse physical strength.

- Use suitable surfaces when riding. Vary the surfaces used and ride in different types of terrain.

- Horses need regular free movement and 'playtime'. Time in the field and going on a walker are likely to be beneficial.

- Feeding: don't overfeed; an overweight horse puts unnecessary load on the joints and is at increased risk of metabolic syndrome which, in turn, increases the risk of laminitis.

Lecture International Society of Equitation Science Congress Uppsala 2010

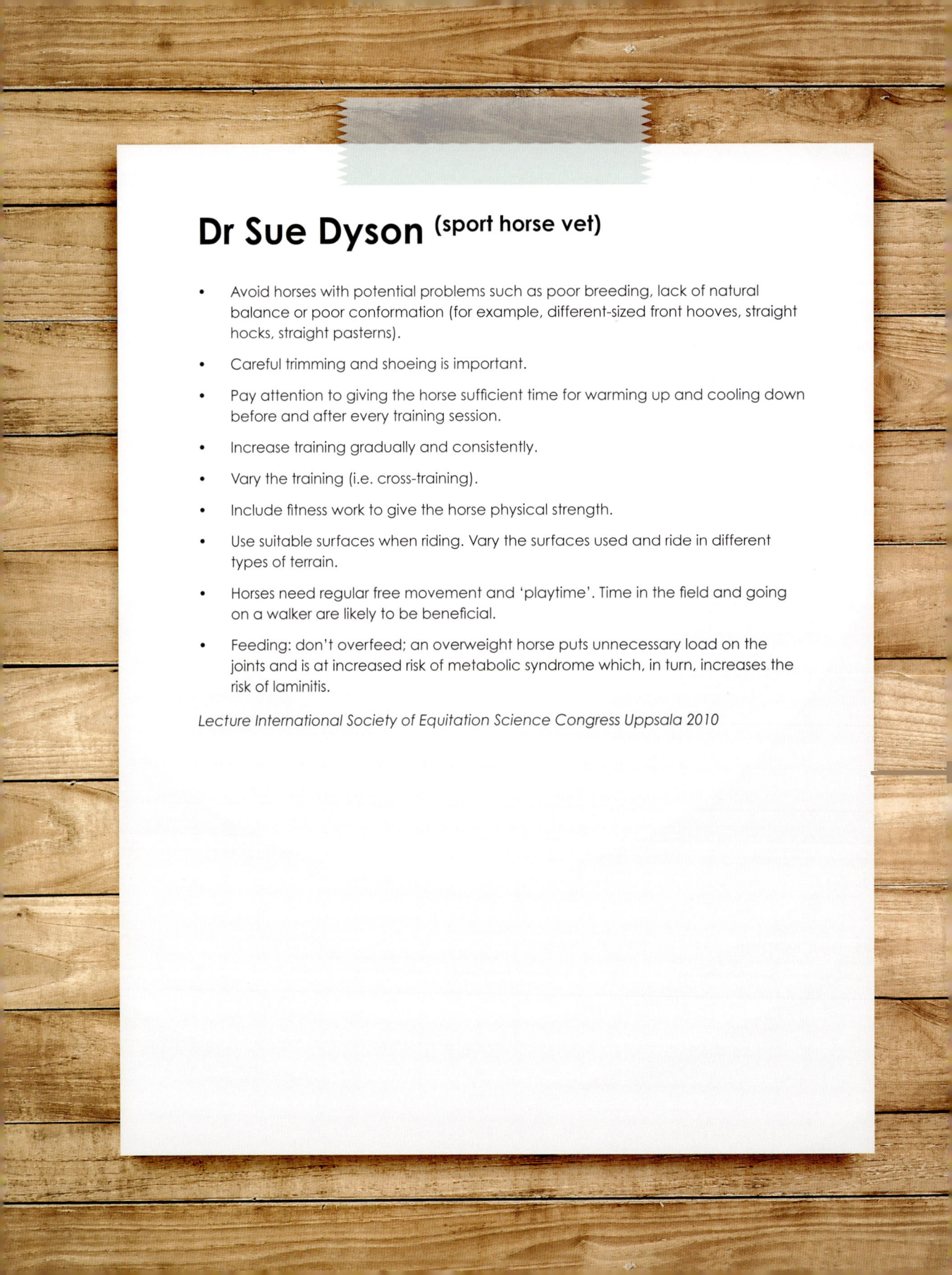

Yogi Breisner (eventing)

- Number one is the horse's conformation, and that he has a natural balance and is light on his feet. A bit also that he has an inborn will to work and to keep fit. Conformation is especially about how he stands on his legs. A horse who is a bit straight in his pasterns and has a straight shoulder will tend to be more predisposed to injury. But there are, of course, individual differences, so horses who have correct conformation may get injured anyway, and the other way around.

- Number two is the training, to develop the horse's balance and get him to use his body in the right way. The horse needs to build strength in his body so that he carries himself and does not put unnecessary load on his legs. Among human athletes there are none who do not work on their strength and fitness besides their primary sport. This is something the horse also needs. One exercise is to work with cavalletti (ride over six poles with three repetitions) and hill training, up and down inclines – that I think is important and good. I also think it is a good exercise for the horse to walk on the side of a hill.

- Choose the riding surface in training. Do not do a lot of work on hard surfaces, and not so much on sand-based mixtures with wax or fibre, which gives a lot of grip. You want a bit of 'give' for the hoof. Personally, I think there is nothing better than a good grass surface. Roadwork is an old British tradition when you walk and trot to build up the horse over a period of six to eight weeks. But if you trot a lot on tarmac it will result in wear and tear, so it is a sensitive balance.

- Be careful with the young horse. He is still developing physically and the skeleton will not be fully matured until the horse is about seven years old.

- General management; shoeing, feeding and that you learn to read the horse's signals so that you can adjust the training to how well or not he is feeling.

- Make a well-thought out competition plan. How many competitions? Where?

Interview November 2015

4. The Right Horse
– are you a good match?

'Reflect on what level of training and experience you are at now, and get an honest outside opinion. Look for a horse who is suitable, preferably a schoolmaster if you do not have previous experience of educating a younger horse.'

Equine insurance expert Dr Charlie Lindberg and equine behaviour researcher Dr Malin Axel-Nilsson

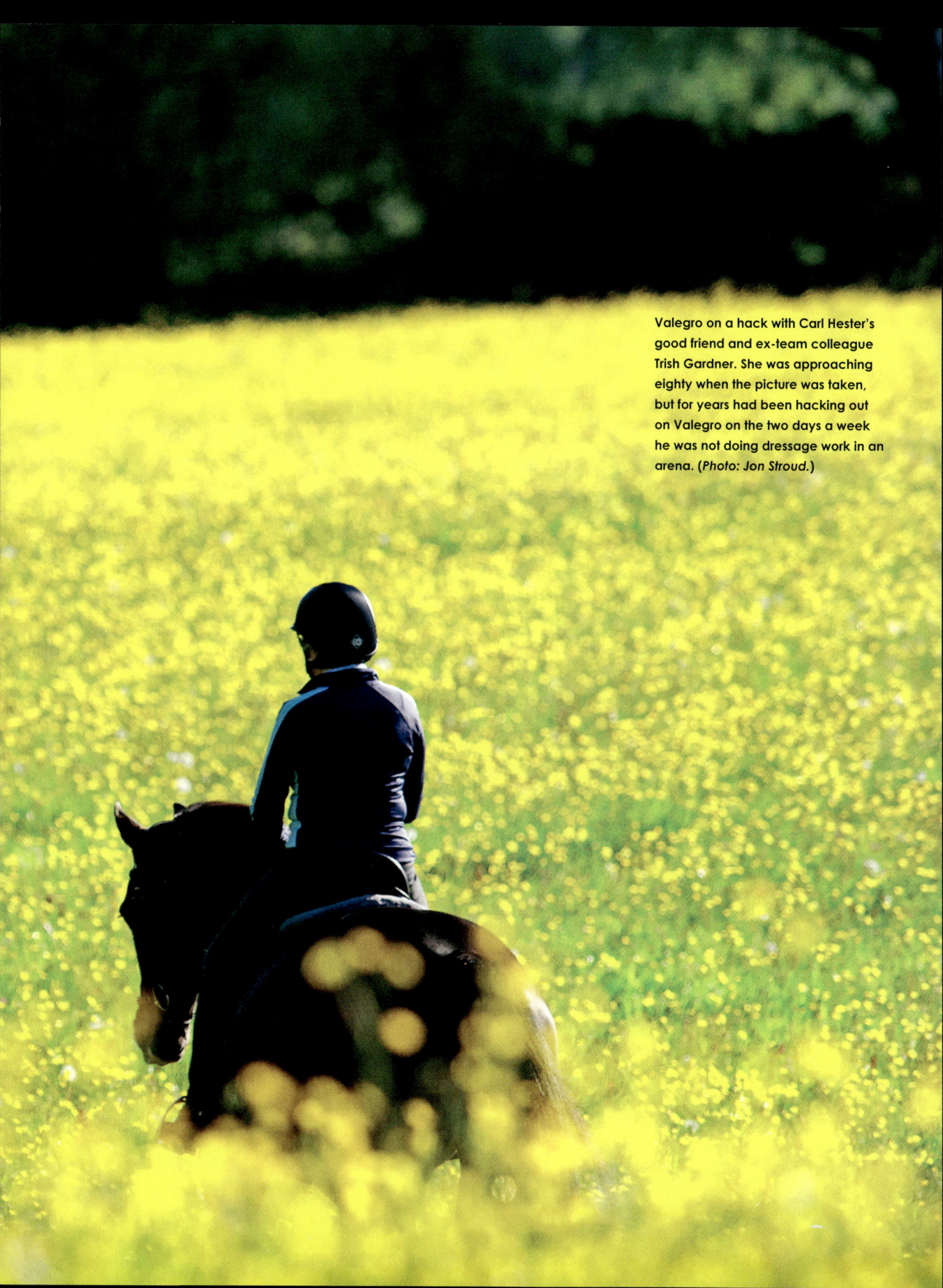

Valegro on a hack with Carl Hester's good friend and ex-team colleague Trish Gardner. She was approaching eighty when the picture was taken, but for years had been hacking out on Valegro on the two days a week he was not doing dressage work in an arena. (*Photo: Jon Stroud.*)

SPORT HORSE SOUNDNESS AND PERFORMANCE

Matchmaking tour

As Dr Charlie Lindberg indicates in his list of horse buying advice at the end of this chapter, the Swedish equine insurance company AGRIA has found rider-horse compatibility very important for horse longevity.

In January 2017 they organised a lecture tour on that subject, simply titled 'Matchmaking', covering Sweden from north to south. One of the speakers was Dr Malin Axel-Nilsson, quoted above, and there were equine vets, a lawyer and top riders.

When the US won Olympic gold at Athens in 2004, Beezie Madden's team-mate was Peter Wylde. He gives the same advice as equine insurance vet Charlie Lindberg; that the rider who goes to try a new horse should not only analyse the horse, but first make an honest appraisal of themselves as a rider. What are your own weaknesses and strengths, and how is that likely to affect your relationship with this particular horse? The legendary dressage ace Kyra Kyrklund also makes that point later on in this chapter.

To succeed in equestrian sport you need a plan, as in most endeavours. The importance of a plan is stressed by former World Champion Franke Sloothaak, among others.

The first step is finding the right horse for you, including the point that you make a good match together.

In Sweden and some other countries a lot of focus in buying horses is on flexion tests and X-rays at the vet inspection. While several of the experts quoted stress that you should avoid buying a horse with problems, by 'the right horse' they also mean 'right' in a wider context. This includes analysing what is not obvious right now but can give early warning of problems ahead.

- The horse's conformation, with any weak spots that can affect both soundness and rideability.
- Breeding (sire and dam, bloodlines), that for the expert also can give hints about both rideability and how strong or fragile the horse is.
- How was the horse raised (as a foal/youngster).
- Temperament and attitude to work – and simply if you 'click'.

POINTS TO CONSIDER

Conformation

Beezie Madden's first advice concerning horses and soundness is the theme of this chapter; choosing the right horse, paying close attention to conformation and getting a thorough vet inspection. Famous sport horse vet Dr Sue Dyson has also stressed the importance of conformation and that you should be careful in your choice of horse if you want long-term soundness.

Conformation can in effect also affect rideability. One example is a horse built 'downhill', who is likely to be heavier on the forehand.

Some 2,400 years ago, in the first known handbook on horses and riding, the Greek cavalry officer Xenophon warned against buying horses with conformational weaknesses such as straight pasterns or weak hocks, as experience had shown that increased the risk of unsoundness. He recommended choosing horses with lots of bone, which traditionally has been associated with soundness.

Genetics/parentage

Horse people often discuss horse breeding; the sire and dam. Bloodlines are traditionally linked to both talent and soundness. Certain bloodlines are sometimes said to produce more fragile or sounder horses than others. Traditional advice is against breeding from injury-prone horses (which is, in reality, often ignored when breeding from mares after an injury or from stallions with short competition careers). At the same time an association between genetics and soundness has now been demonstrated through scientific research. Analysis of data from tests on Swedish Warmblood four-year-olds showed that certain stallions produced, for example, progeny with a higher propensity than others for poor hoof quality. Scientists have found certain genes that indicate that a horse is more disposed to, for example, stress fractures, osteochondrosis (OCD), or navicular disease syndrome. What you can do as a buyer, as insurance vet Charlie Lindberg advises later on in this chapter, is to ask questions about the horse's background.

How was the horse raised?

Former World Champion Franke Sloothaak has stressed that, when getting a new horse in his yard, he makes a point of finding out as much as possible about how the horse was

SPORT HORSE SOUNDNESS AND PERFORMANCE

The traditional view in horse breeding is that young horses should be kept with other youngsters of the same age and sex, in a herd and given plenty of pasture space to play and run about, preferably on undulating ground. Research now supports the thought that early, natural exercise promotes the body's adaptation to later work. *(Photo: Roland Thunholm.)*

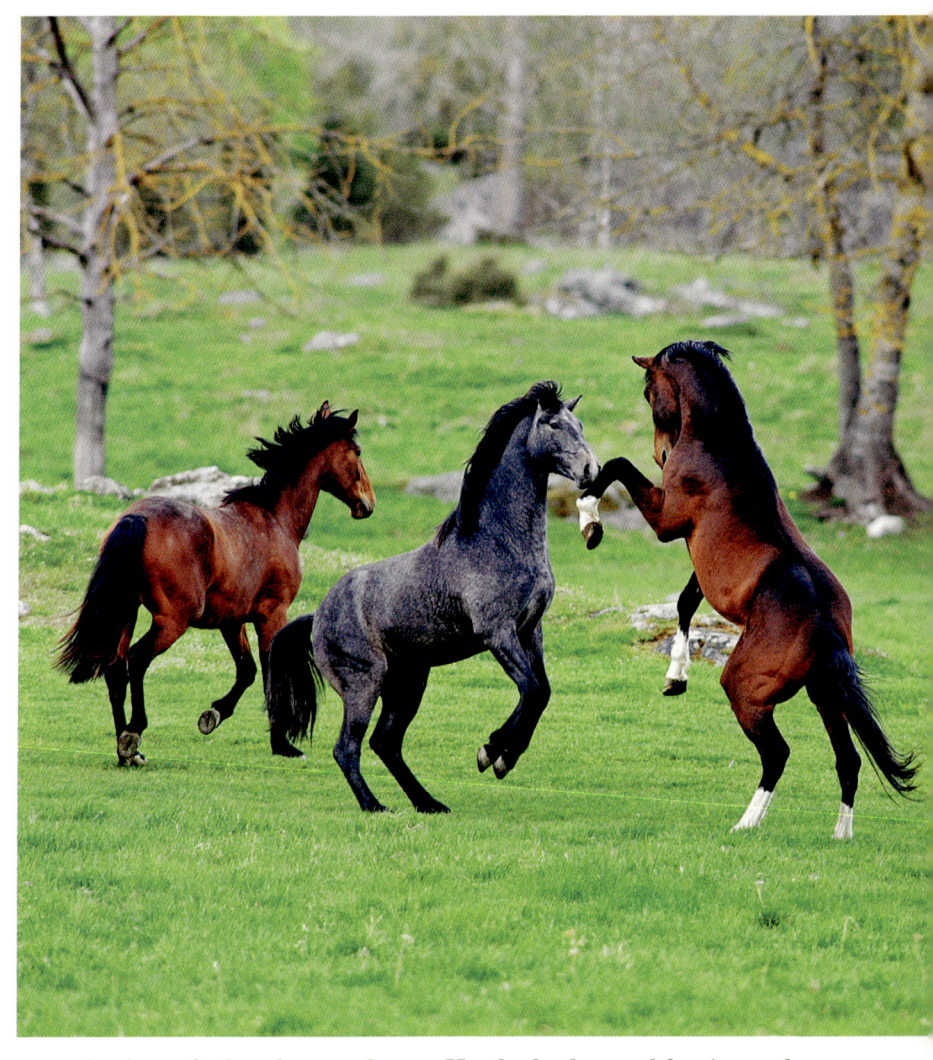

raised as a foal and young horse. Has he had a good farrier and received correct hoof trimming; has he been wormed properly; has he been fed correctly? There is a traditional view that how a young horse is raised can affect his long-term soundness. Among factors recommended is that of keeping youngsters together in herds, on large and preferably undulating pasture, so that the young horse gets the chance of plenty and varied

THE RIGHT HORSE – ARE YOU A GOOD MATCH?

Young horses need to play and run

It would be a major scientific challenge to evaluate the traditional view that how a young horse is raised can affect soundness in the long term, not least as the horses being studied would need to be followed for years, to find out if they stay sound or not. But a few years ago equine vets from the veterinary faculty in Utrecht performed a ground-breaking study testing more immediate effects of exercise or lack thereof on foals and yearlings, including being out at pasture. At the EEHNC* on the health and feeding of sport horses in Bruges 2015, Dr Harold Brommer from the Utrecht group pointed out that the joint cartilage in a newborn foal needs to be 'primed' through the foal moving about, in order for the cartilage to respond to loading and to develop properly. Such priming will be finished by more than two-thirds by the time the foal is six months old, almost completely when the horse is two years old, and fully when the horse is four years old. After four years of age the cartilage cells will become less active.

When foals and yearlings play and run about this means that their body gets signals to adapt to exercise. The Dutch study had three groups of foals. One group was kept with their dams in stables from birth, one group was kept out on pasture and a third group was kept in the stable but had daily canter exercise on a track. Simply put, the foals who were kept in stables and thus without exercise had a poorer development of, for example, joint cartilage and bone.

*European Equine Health and Nutrition Congress; organised in Belgium and held every second year. Open not only to scientists but also other horse industry professionals.

Better conformation = better career longevity

Research at the Swedish University of Agricultural Sciences has shown that horses with good marks for conformation at the quality testing of four-year-olds had, as a mean, longer competition careers than those with poorer marks for conformation. Associations between certain conformational weaknesses and risk of injury have been shown also in Thoroughbred racehorses.

natural exercise. Before the era of mineral supplements, lime-rich land (where the grass contained lime) was regarded as good for horse breeding as it helped develop strong bone.

As a horse buyer you can ask the same questions as Franke Sloothaak in his analysis, especially if it is a young horse in question, and not imported. Keep a sceptical mind! Was the horse bred by a first-time breeder who kept the foal alone with the dam in a small paddock at home, or was he brought up at a stud in a professional environment?

ARE YOU A GOOD MATCH?

Breeding, conformation and how the horse was raised can be suspected to affect soundness. But how the future career of the horse will work out is also determined by the rider. It is important that the horse has a character/personality and a level of experience that fits your profile as a rider. How and whether a horse and rider fit together is sometimes as instant as the chemistry between two people, but the experience of each also needs to match. Xenophon recommended 2,400 years ago that an amateur owner should not attempt to train a young horse, but should send the horse to a professional (and spell out carefully in a contract what the horse should have learnt when returning!). Fitting the right horse with the right rider is often also a question of safety, and potentially of soundness. If, for example, you feel nervous about going out hacking because the horse is more spooky or more 'explosive' than you are comfortable with, it will be difficult to get the variation in training which champion riders recommended in the previous chapter.

Beezie Madden's husband, John Madden, a top coach and dealer, pointed out in an interview that it is important that you like your horse as a 'person'. If you are going to work with a horse every day without a natural liking for him, it is more difficult to get good results.

Franke Sloothaak also pointed out that you must realise that the perfect horse with no faults does not exist, just as the perfect rider or human does not exist. If you have bought a horse who you soon realise is not right for you, you should either give up straight away and sell him on, or be prepared to put work in if you cannot afford to find another one, Franke said.

In Sweden, where this book was first released, there are consumer laws that are very generous to the buyer, but not necessarily in the interest of the horse. They allow a buyer to make mistakes with the horse and yet demand to have the deal cancelled even two years later.

If you find that you and a horse do not make a good match there is no shame in that. There are plenty of examples of famous riders who said 'no' to horses, who then went on to have great success with another top rider. There are also examples of famous horse and rider combinations where the riders first thought they had a problem but in the end had great success with the same horse. Olympic champion Eric Lamaze and Hickstead are one example – the stallion was a very difficult ride when Lamaze first had him, but they became world-beaters together. We are, of course, talking here about super-talented riders whose profession is to be able to ride almost any horse, and who spend their working days doing that. For someone who does not ride full-time and only has one or two horses, and maybe gets their own horse for the very first time, it is both easier and more enjoyable if the horse and rider 'fit' right from the start.

Apart from considering temperament and rideability it is also important to be honest with yourself whether your physical talent fits the horse's. There is not much point in choosing a horse with, for example, spectacular gaits or huge scope over fences, if you have to struggle to follow the movement or to stay on over the fence.

Franke Sloothaak and Kyra Kyrklund on trying a horse to buy

Franke Sloothaak has the following to say about trying a horse:

'Get up on the horse and reflect on what feeling you get. Sometimes you get a good feeling when getting up on a horse for the first time. If things do not feel right straight from the beginning there is no point in staying on.

The things you do not like the first time you get on a horse will not change. People think they can change a horse, but he will keep his nature from when he is four or five years old. He can get more muscled, he can learn, become better schooled and get more experience, but fundamentally he will be the same horse.

Kyra Kyrklund has also pointed out the importance of first impressions in the saddle. In parallel with Peter Wylde's comments elsewhere in the book she adds that it is important to reflect on your own weaknesses as a rider in relation to the horse's.

'Concentrate on the horse; on what feeling you are getting. The purpose of trying the horse is, after all, not to impress any bystanders. It is to get a feel of this horse; to find out whether you will make a good match and suit each other, Kyra said at a clinic together with Franke at Göteborg Horse Show in Sweden. Always have in mind what your weaknesses are as a rider and whether the horse's strengths compensate for that, and the other way around. When buying a horse always also try to take into account that the horse's strengths compensate for your weakness, and the other way around.'

Kyra continued: 'I am, for example, much better at trot work than canter. Therefore I prefer to have horses who have a naturally good and easy canter, as I prefer to be trotting and work on that gait.' Kyra also gave the advice never to fully trust a video of a horse.

Champions are not born ready-made – they are brought on

As is clear from the examples above, top horses do not become world-beaters on their own. Former World Champion Jos Lansink has said that you have to shape and develop the horse, He mentions as an example the four horses in the individual final of the 2006 World Championships, that he won: his own Cumano, Pialotta (Edwina Tops-Alexander, previously ridden by Rolf Göran Bengtsson and Steve Guerdat), Shutterfly (Meredith Michaels-Beerbaum) and Authentic (Beezie Madden). None of those were obvious World Champion medallists when they were youngsters, Jos said. He went on:

'But they must have quality from the start. A good balance is one of the most important traits one is looking for, and that shows in loose jumping. In loose jumping you can also spot scope, but a super-careful horse (as in not wanting to touch fences) might not jump so high in loose jumping. A careful horse needs support from the rider.'

Other riders or showjumping enthusiasts might sometimes say that a certain champion rider is 'lucky' to ride a certain horse. But insiders are more likely think that the horse was lucky to get the right (in effect, skilled and with a lot of feel) rider. This is a comment made by the professional riders who had Zenith as a young horse, before he was bought for Jeroen Dubbeldam and won double gold medals both at the World Equestrian Games in 2014 and the Europeans in 2015. Jeroen was lucky to get Zenith, but Zenith is a sensitive horse and was lucky to come to Jeroen, Zenith's discoverer and part-owner Dutch horse dealer Willy van der Ham said. The sensitive Warum Nicht with Isabell Werth is another such example, their trainer Wolfram Wittig has said:

'In the beginning people asked why we even bought him. It worked, but only with Isabell in the saddle'. He is a fighter, absolutely, but he needed a leader. He needed Isabell.'

SPORT HORSE SOUNDNESS AND PERFORMANCE

For Rodrigo Pessoa it was not love at first sight when he first tried Baloubet du Rouet as a young horse. But his father Neco saw the potential in the chestnut stallion who, when more mature, won Olympic gold and three World Cup Finals. For a non-professional who is buying their own horse it is important to find a horse you really get on with straight away. (Nelson Pessoa also predicted years ahead that Baloubet would be a top breeding sire, and he was right on that score, too). (Photo: Roland Thunholm.)

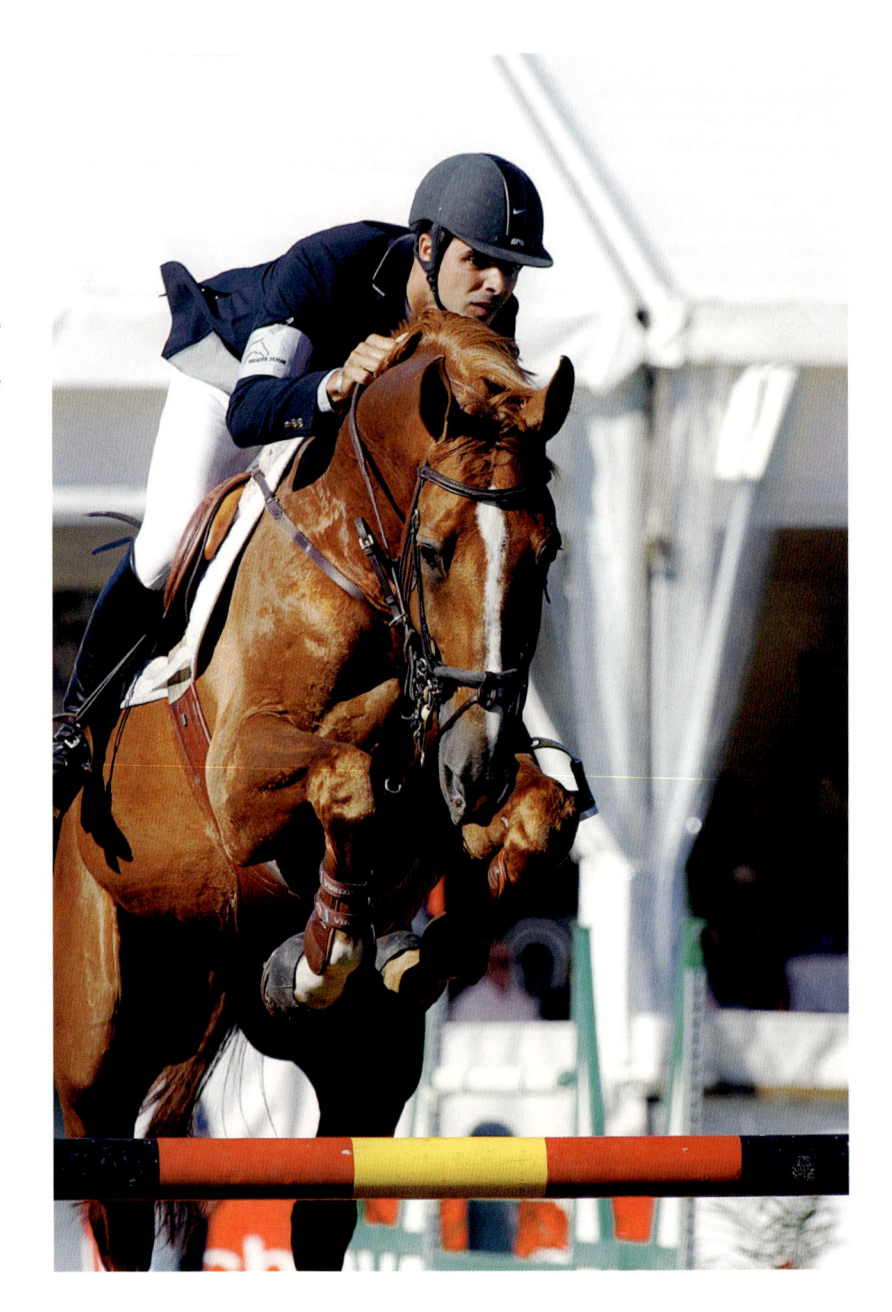

'That the horse and rider make a good match is important for the well-being of the horse.'

There is increasing focus on scientific study of horse behaviour and welfare, including at the Swedish University of Agricultural Sciences.

'Consider carefully what you want to do with your horse; concentrate on how it feels when you ride and handle him and try several different horses before buying.' This advice about buying horses was given by Dr Malin Axel-Nilsson in her doctoral thesis presented in the autumn of 2015. She wants to underline the importance of having realistic ambitions when buying a horse and, like insurance vet Dr Charlie Lindberg at the end of this chapter, gives the advice to get input from coaches and other knowledgeable persons, who can give a more objective view of your scope as a rider, and of the temperament of both you and the horse.' Sadly it happens that riders buy horses that really do not suit them. Most people, of course, have dreams of what the horse should be capable of – for example, in showjumping – that not always are realistic or achievable', she said.

Modern sport horse breeding has resulted in horses who are more sensitive and lively than those bred in the past for the cavalry or farm work. Today's horses have a lot more natural talent for the sport, but in many cases their talent requires an experienced rider. This is not always obvious at the first test ride.

'The price of mistakes in horse buying is eventually paid by the horse and this is unfortunate', Malin Axel-Nilsson said in an interview. Her advice about repeated 'dates' echoes the advice by Dr Charlie Lindberg 'That the horse and rider make a good match is important for the well-being and welfare of the horse, for the safety of the rider and to get the best possible performance', Malin Axel-Nilsson said.

Malin specifically warned riders not to buy a young horse if they had not already had previous experience of training young horses.

Her Ph.D research included mental tests of a group of horses at the National Equestrian Centre at Flyinge. They were faced with a number of challenges, such as being left alone in an unfamiliar stable and approaching unfamiliar objects in an indoor arena, such as open umbrellas, that could be perceived as frightening. The tests were standard in equine behavioural research.

Study riders were also classified based on personality profiles into 'emotionally stable' or more unstable, that is, in simple terms, more 'chilled' or more anxious.

'We found that some of the horses were quite easy to handle while others became both more explosive and negatively affected by the challenges. Riders with a more cool temperament had a better feel with the more explosive horses than the other way around. Riders with a more anxious temperament felt more comfortable with the horses who were more calm and independent', Malin said.

SPORT HORSE SOUNDNESS AND PERFORMANCE

Was it love at first sight or the first try?

Rodrigo Pessoa and Baloubet du Rouet
(won three World Cup Finals and individual Olympic gold)

'I had already had about five or six horses by Baloubet's sire Galoubet, and was not overly impressed by this last one. Sure, Baloubet had scope, but I thought "Oh, well, not another Galoubet (son) who is hot and runs to the fence".'

'He said "What a s**t horse"', Rodrigo's father Nelson 'Neco' Pessoa disclosed in a profile about the famous stallion, 'But that was many years ago, when Rodrigo himself was young and used to older horses. If Rodrigo were to see such a youngster today he would also realise what it could become.'

Rodrigo gives his father the honour of realising Baloubet's potential. The first years of Baloubet's career they both competed on him.

Beat Mändli and Ideo du Thot
(World Cup Champions 2007)

'The feeling that he had a good head for jumping I had straight away, but everything else was not quite as I wanted it, for example the mouth was not so good. I said to Rolf Theiler (Ideo's owner) that we will see how it works out', Beat Mändli recalled about his first try on Ideo du Thot at the end of 2004. Mr Theiler had secured the horse for Beat without him trying Ideo first. Ideo had top French bloodlines for jumping and huge scope, but also plenty of surplus energy and some rideability issues. A little more than two years later they won the World Cup Final at Las Vegas.

'I knew quite quickly what he needed. It included flatwork, experience from competitions and improved physical strength. I also felt that I must not do too much too soon but give him time. It is only now that he has become really mature and strong. He is careful, has scope and so on. He has a lot of energy and never tires, that is both a plus and a minus. It is needed in a place like Aachen where they have to jump big courses several days in a row, but he easily gets overconfident, wants a bit too much, and that is not always so easy to handle', Mändli said after their World Cup title in 2007.

Karin Rehbein and Donnerhall
(two World Championship team golds, European team gold, European and World individual bronze)

'He was thin and rangy, but you could tell he had potential. You can feel that straight away', Karin Rehbein said of the stallion when he was four. He had already been second in the 90-day stallion test at Adelheidsdorf, with top marks for rideability. Donnerhall did Medium classes at six and the small tour at seven, but by then could already do Grand Prix movements.

Isabell Werth and Warum Nicht
(World Cup Champions 2007)

'You must come and see him. I think he could be a world-class horse.' This was Isabell Werth's evaluation on the mobile to her horse owner Madeleine Winter-Schulze after being shown a large, gangly son of Weltmeyer at the warm-up in Verden. It was Warum Nicht ('Why Not'), at seven years old.

When Isabell spots a new horse she either gets a 'wow' feeling, or not. With Warum Nicht she immediately thought 'Wow, what a talent'. He was a good model, with a large frame and big movement. He could, at the same time, do with a bit more muscle and he was easily frightened, but Isabell was convinced about his potential and prepared to spend the time to let him develop. In the beginning he was very spooky: he could spook at anything, whether a flower or a shadow. His maternal grandsire Wenzel was known to produce spooky offspring. It was because of that, when Warum Nicht was a youngster, people asked the previous owner: 'How can you buy a foal by Weltmeyer and Wenzel I?' and he replied 'Warum Nicht' in German, and so the horse was named.

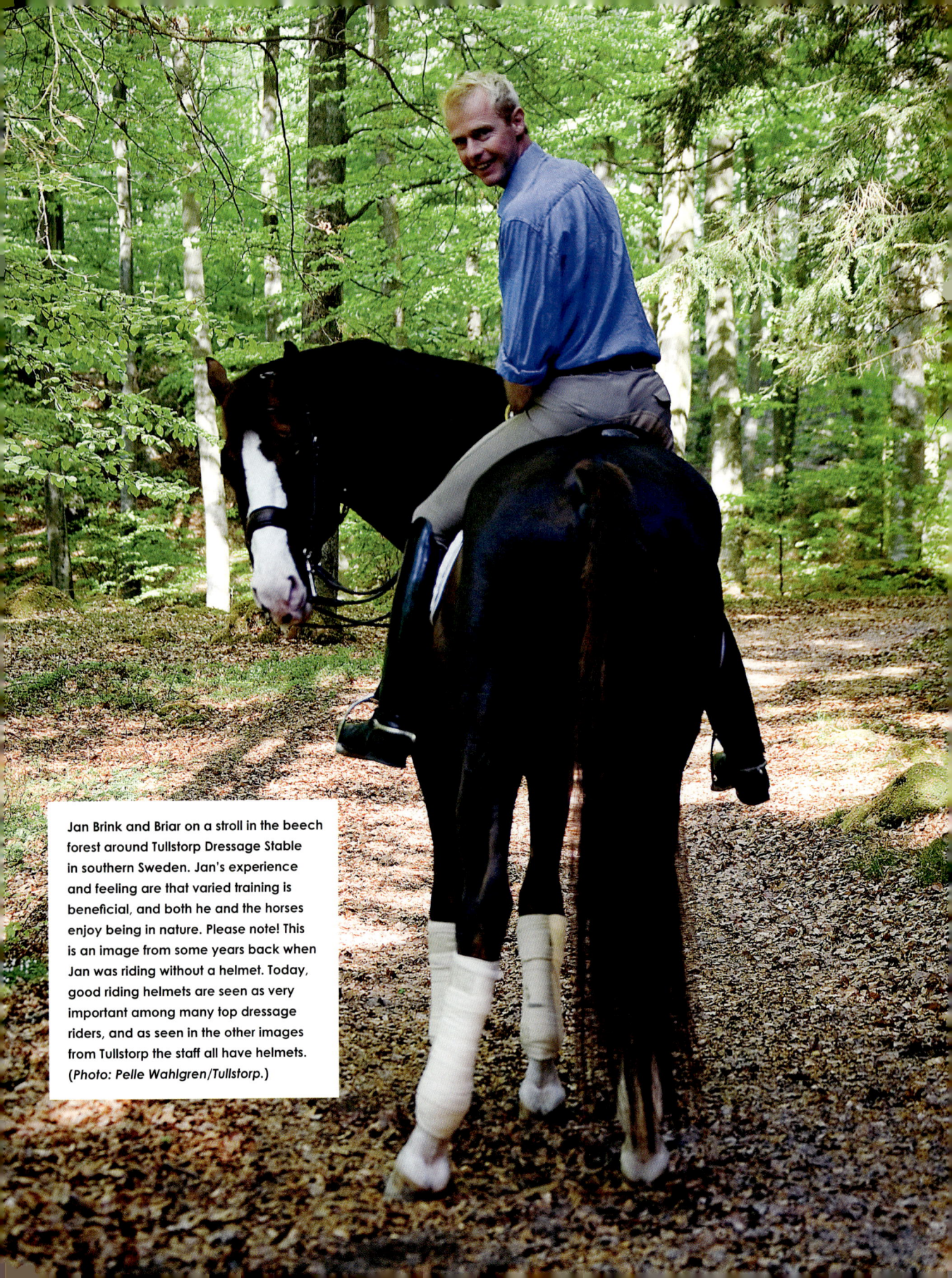

Jan Brink and Briar on a stroll in the beech forest around Tullstorp Dressage Stable in southern Sweden. Jan's experience and feeling are that varied training is beneficial, and both he and the horses enjoy being in nature. Please note! This is an image from some years back when Jan was riding without a helmet. Today, good riding helmets are seen as very important among many top dressage riders, and as seen in the other images from Tullstorp the staff all have helmets. (*Photo: Pelle Wahlgren/Tullstorp.*)

Advice when buying a horse

This advice was kindly provided by top insurance vet Dr Charlie Lindberg.

1. Reflect on what level of training and experience you are at now, and get an honest outside opinion. Look for a horse who is suitable for that level, preferably a schoolmaster if you do not have previous experience of educating a younger horse.
2. Take advice from an experienced horse person. Ask them or your coach/riding teacher to come with you when trying the horse.
3. Try the horse on several occasions and preferably in different environments.
4. Check the background of the horse: breeder, where and how the horse was raised as a youngster, where he was first broken and trained, any competition results. This is easiest with a horse who was bred in your own country, or was imported as a young horse. Different national equestrian federations offer different level of access to competition records.
5. If the horse is insured, ask the owner/vendor for access to insurance records, including any previous veterinary claims. This includes checking that the horse does not have or will get any exclusions on his insurance as a result of previous injury/disease. That can otherwise cause unpleasant surprises when you want to set up your insurance. Do not go through with the deal before the horse's current insurer has been contacted.
6. Have a vet in whom you have confidence to check the horse, and do not let the seller choose. Your own vet is likely to be able to recommend a colleague, if the horse is in a different part of the country. Try to be present during the inspection.
7. Agree beforehand with the seller who will pay for the inspection, for X-rays, ultrasound or other additional testing. If the deal does not go through, who will pay what?
8. Set up a detailed sale agreement.
9. Different countries have different rules on buyers' guarantees for horses, including those based on EU rules. One recommendation is not to change the insurer or type of insurance, but stay with the same company for at least as long as the buyer's guarantee holds and make sure that the insurance company covers the risk. The horse will then have insurance protection, which is important for any hidden faults.
10. If you have any doubts about the deal because of what the vet's report said, what you yourself have felt when trying the horse, or because of what competition records show, maybe those doubts will stay with you – do not buy that horse!
11. And finally: sell the horse if you realise he does not suit you! If you bought a horse who proved to be unsuitable it is wise to sell him on and buy a different horse, who fits better with what you want. Trying to get the previous owner to take a horse back can be both expensive and troublesome.

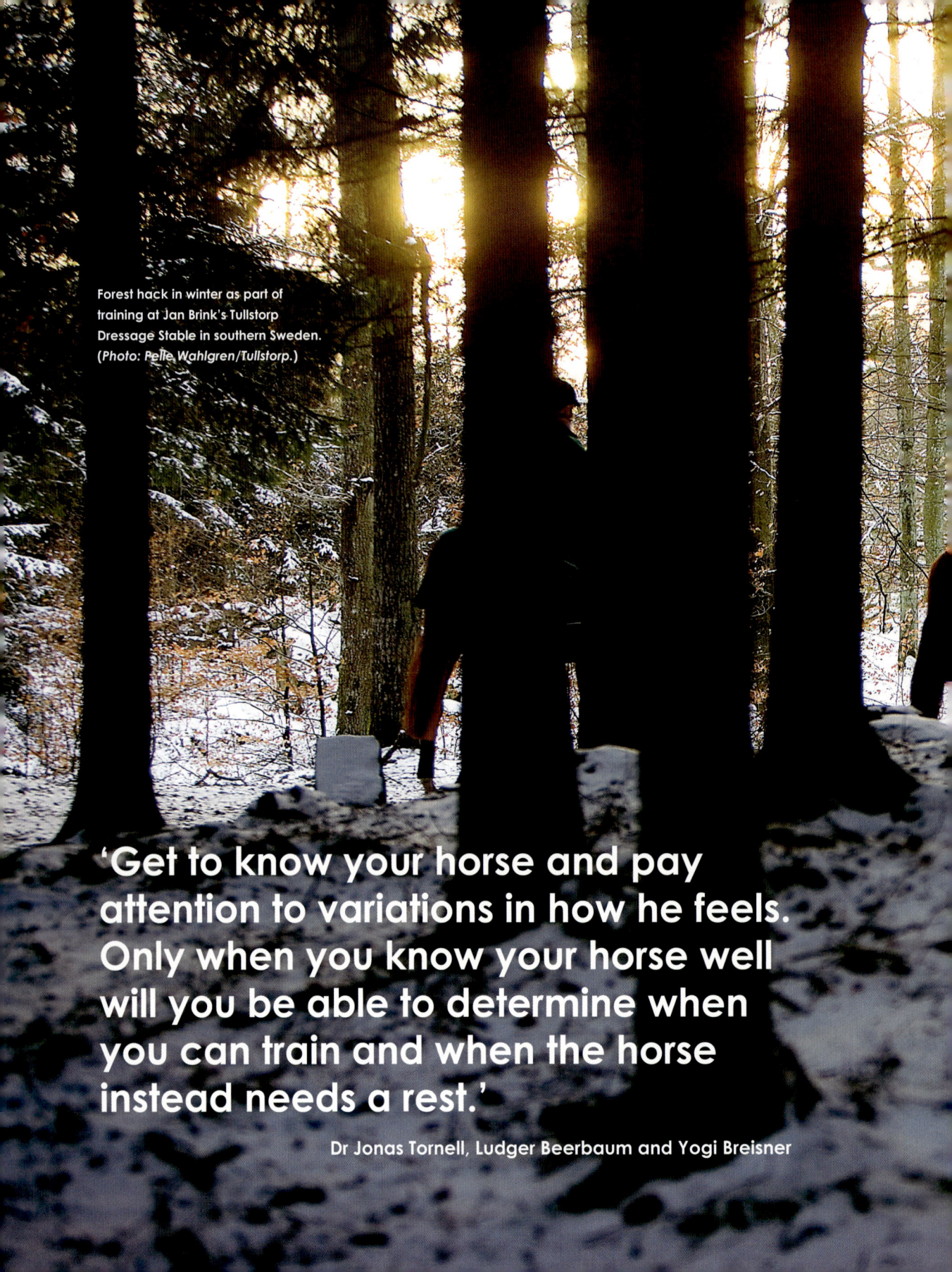

Forest hack in winter as part of training at Jan Brink's Tullstorp Dressage Stable in southern Sweden. (*Photo: Pelle Wahlgren/Tullstorp.*)

'Get to know your horse and pay attention to variations in how he feels. Only when you know your horse well will you be able to determine when you can train and when the horse instead needs a rest.'

Dr Jonas Tornell, Ludger Beerbaum and Yogi Breisner

5. Allow your horse time

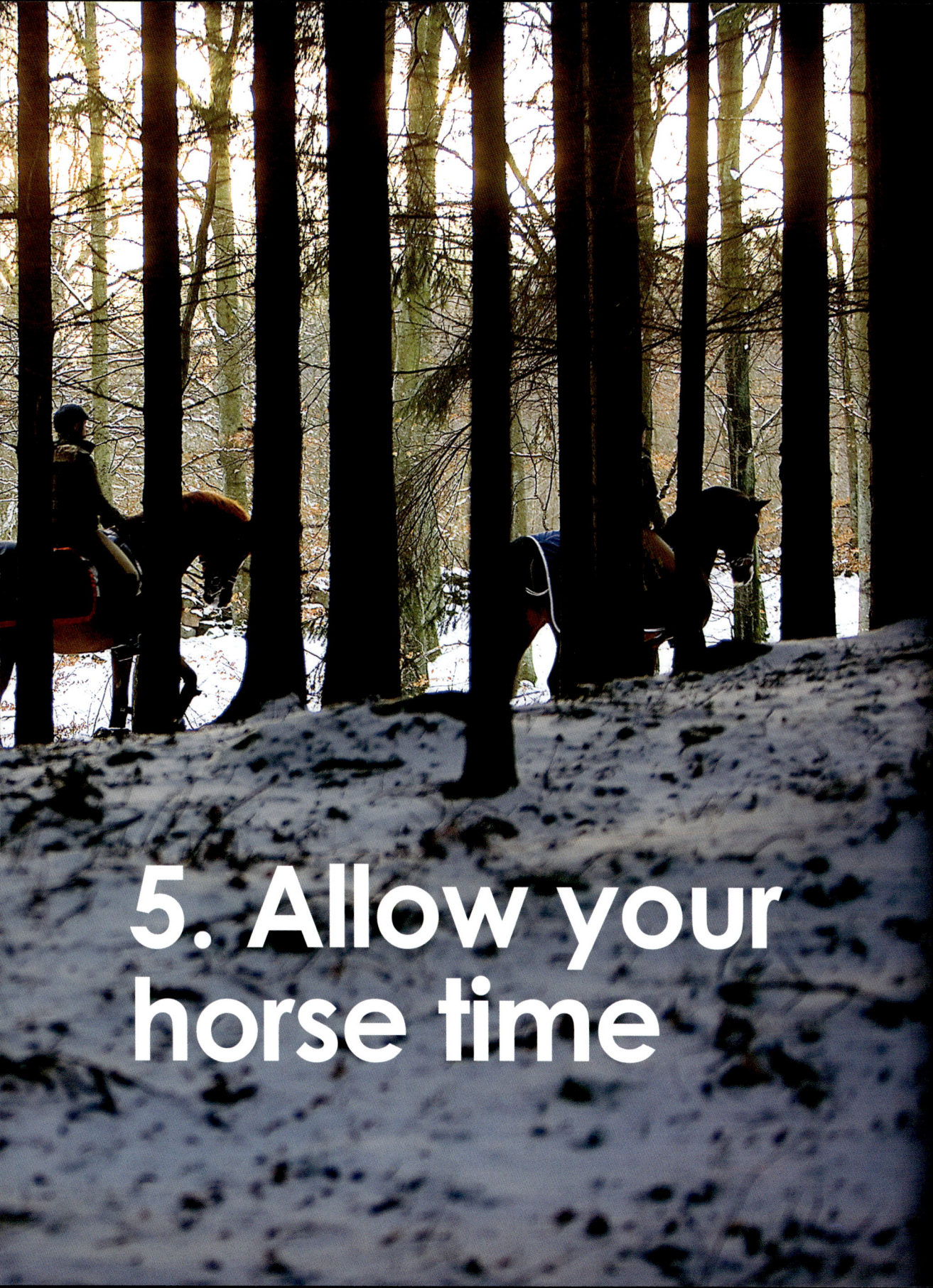

Give the horse time to adapt!

A very clear example that a new horse needs time to adapt to his new job after being sold is provided by data from a study on riding school horses at the Swedish University of Agricultural Sciences.

Riding schools with few orthopaedic injuries (measured as veterinary insurance claims) as a mean had at least eleven weeks gradual introduction to lessons for new horses (and some up to one year).

In contrast, riding schools with a very high level of orthopaedic injuries (measured as veterinary insurance claims) had, in several cases, no introduction time but let new horses do full work straight away.

These results indicate that horses need time to physically adapt to riding school work, and work at the specific riding school. This was irrespective of the horse's general fitness.

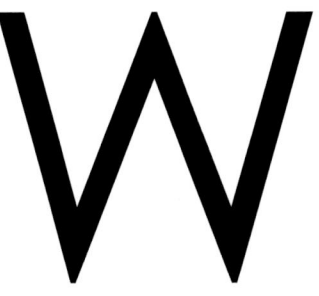

When the new horse has arrived it is important that you take your time to get to know him. Give him time to get used to his new surroundings and routines, and adapt physically to his new job. We will come back to why the horse needs time for physical adaptation in Chapter 9 on training.

'It is sadly extremely common that the rider does not have enough sense or enough feel not to ask more from the horse than his current level of training allows without overstrain', Professor Gerhard Forsell said in 1927 in connection with preventing injury in young horses.

Getting to know the horse and allowing time for adaptation comes first in jumping legend Ludger Beerbaum's bullet point advice on soundness in Chapter 3. Former World Champion Jos Lansink makes the same point:

'One problem when an owner sends a horse to us is that he wants quick results. But in my opinion it takes a year before you have learnt all the "buttons" in a horse and know each other completely. If a horse is new in the yard we begin by giving him time, letting him get a feel of the place and relax. Then we start building him up and take one step at a time. If you give them a bit of time you can get better results in the long term. It is also a question of the horse's background, what he has done earlier.'

Later on in the book I discuss how the body 'reconstructs' itself in response to work and training, a process that takes months. One important point is that the horse also needs time to adapt to a different rider. A different rider means different work for the horse, because every rider sits differently and makes different demands.

Horse vets quite often see injuries and physical problems in horses about half a year after they have changed hands (or rather rider). This can be interpreted as indicating that the new rider has wanted to do too much too soon (note Ludger Beerbaum's bullet point advice in Chapter 3), in relation to how much the horse's body has had the chance to adapt to the new work.

SHOW THE YOUNG HORSE RESPECT

Shortly after Jos Lansink won the 2006 World Championships he met Swedish juniors and Young Riders for a seminar at an international show in Linköping. One point on the agenda was educating young horses. He underlined the importance of a young horse not getting any bad experiences, and indirectly advised young riders against trying to develop a young horse on their own. Lansink employs young stable riders, but they are not allowed to go to a show on their own with young horses. Jos said it is very important that both have supervision from the ground, as with young riders and young horses a lot can happen. One traditional strategy of developing young horses is to have periods of training/competition and rest/recovery alternately during the year.

Another piece of advice that has been offered by both Michael Whitaker and Carl Hester is to let the especially nervous and sensitive young horse come along with an older horse in the lorry or trailer, to a show, put the tack on and ride him around a bit and then let him go home again without competing (remember to check with the organiser beforehand). The horse thus gets a chance to get used to the show atmosphere without the stress of competing. One example of that is Carl's top horse Nip Tuck who travelled with groom Alan Davies for three years without showing, including to the Continent.

You can get a young horse used to new experiences just by bringing him to a different riding centre or arena and ride him there. Another choice, which is basically what Lansink discussed, is to compete to get experience, without riding to win.

Jos Lansink's schedule for young horses

Six years: They usually compete through September. Then they get three months in the field and then they are started again when they have turned seven. They need some breaks.

When Jos was stable jockey at the Zangersheide Stud for about eight years he used to help measure young horses, and saw that a six-year-old could grow 3–4cm in a year. Then they need extra time, and that is good mentally as well. Twelve months of competition is too much for any horse. It is important to have a plan and choose the competitions.

Seven years: Varies with the horse. They get further breaks from competition, but not as long as three months. The ones who do everything right compete less, but those who are not as good need to get out more in competition. But people often do it the other way around; horses who are not doing so well they leave at home and instead compete with the ones who are good, because that is more fun. But a young horse needs experience in competition. It is easy to think you have a superstar at home, but before he gets out and competes you really know very little about the genuine quality.

Michael Whitaker has said he does not jump his young horses before the basic dressage/flatwork is in place. He points out that it is important not to jump big fences to soon, and to avoid long jumping sessions, so that the horse does not start to have fences down just from being tired. In Chapter 9 on training he also points out that it is important that the horse has first been allowed to build general fitness before being expected to do other work.

TREAT THE HORSE AS AN INDIVIDUAL

It is again very important to emphasise that the rider develops a feel for and 'listens' to the horse. One of the key points of advice from top riders is for riders to try and develop that feel:

1. Understand the personality of the horse and adjust to it.
2. Let the horse tell you what he is ready for.
3. Don't expect too much too soon.
4. Let the horse drop a level (class) or two now and again, both if you are having problems and if he has done very well.

Franke Sloothaak quotes Nelson Pessoa, Rodrigo's father:

'He has put it in a good way; a horse is like a book, and you must start on the first page. Many riders start in the middle, and then they get problems. They do not understand the horse and where the weak points are. Beginning on the first page means that you start by really watching and analysing the horse. Look at his breeding. Consider how that might be reflected in this mentality. Is he hot? Honest? Difficult to ride? That is often linked to the breeding.'

A happy horse performs better!

'I want to underline how important it is that the horse is in a good mood', Franke Sloothaak said. 'You must work on

ALLOW YOUR HORSE TIME

the horse's mentality, encourage his ambition. Horses should be happy, and feel good. They need variety, for example. The horse must want to work on his own account. If he loses interest he needs to rest, and he will tell you that. There your own feel as a rider comes in. It is important that you pay attention to signs that the horse is not feeling well – maybe he is mentally tired, or feels some pain in his body. Then you must let him rest and let the vet examine him. If he hurts somewhere, work is pointless. The horse being healthy and sound is the most important of all.'

Dressage rider Patrik Kittel commented that, in his experience of almost twenty-five years, horses are almost never 'stupid' or 'difficult' as such, but in such cases are signalling pain or that they are being asked more than they are ready for.

The importance of the horse being happy is also emphasised by John Whitaker, Peter Wylde and Malin Baryard-Johnsson. One common thread with these champion riders is their focus on keeping the horse confident, or restoring his confidence if it is lost.

'Just like with children, you should look more at what the horse is doing right, and make him understand that', Peter Wylde said. He went on: 'The reward can be a sugar cube, a pat, a loose rein, and through your body language telling the horse that "this is good".'

Peter Wylde, like Franke Sloothaak, tells riders who want to compete to listen to the horse regarding at what level he

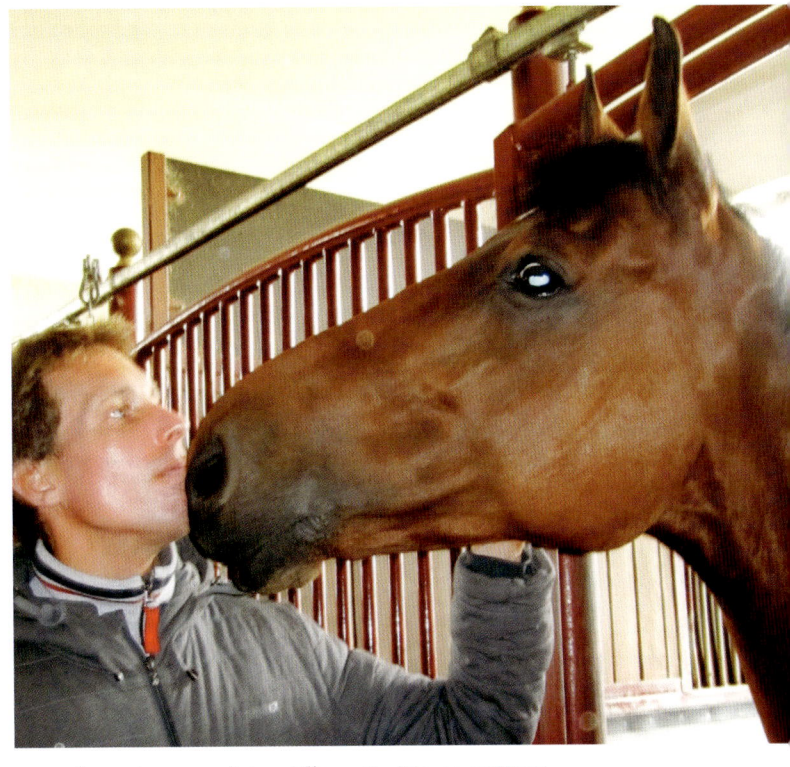

Confidence and trust. Henrik von Eckermann and Cantinero at home at his then boss Ludger Beerbaum's training centre in Riesenbeck in May 2015. Four days after this picture was taken they did a double clear in the Rome Nation's Cup, and two days later again they won the five-star Rome Grand Prix, one of Europe's most prestigious. (Photo: Dr Cecilia Lönnell.)

should do so. This way of thinking is a matter of course for many champion riders. He says:

'The horse tells you what he can do, or not. The results will tell you where you are now. If you are having a fence down, drop a class or two, until the horse finds it easy. There is nothing wrong with riding in small classes and winning the whole time. When you do that well you can aim higher. If you are going clear, that is good. If not, you should take a step downward and analyse what you need to work on, and practise instead of competing. You should face reality. You must understand that you can hurt the horse if you ask too much. You often want a little bit more, but you must realise your responsibility as a rider and what an art it is to adjust the work of the horse.'

Franke agrees: 'Again you should have a plan, but adjust it according to the horse's current form. If, for example, the horse hits very good form and wins something big, but then does not jump as well another week, you should be prepared to let him do a lower class, or scratch him altogether.'

Rolf Göran Bengtsson's very skilled groom, Celia Rintjes, has described how Rolf has sometimes scratched a horse in a class, after walking the course, because he felt the course did not suit the horse at that moment. This applied to young horses.

Franke comments: 'If a horse is feeling really good you can let him do a bigger class than you had planned. If not, he should do a lower class, or maybe not jump at all. Even a horse at Grand Prix level you should sometimes give a lighter job, otherwise you will run out of petrol. If a horse has a fence down in training you need not get worked up about that. The intelligent horse will learn from his mistake. But it can also happen that you, for example, turn too sharp in a jump-off and crash – an accident can happen – but then the horse can lose confidence. This, the rider must realise. The rider must then rewind, and analyse what can be done to help the horse regain his confidence.'

Opposite: When Rolf Göran Bengtsson got the ride on Ninja La Silla he was a useful Nation's Cup horse, but with Rolf developed into one of the best showjumpers in the world. The combination won individual Olympic silver in 2008 and became European Champions in 2011. In addition they were very close to a place in the final four at the 2010 World Equestrian Games. Ninja was sixteen years old when he and Rolf won the Europeans. *(Photo: Roland Thunholm.)*

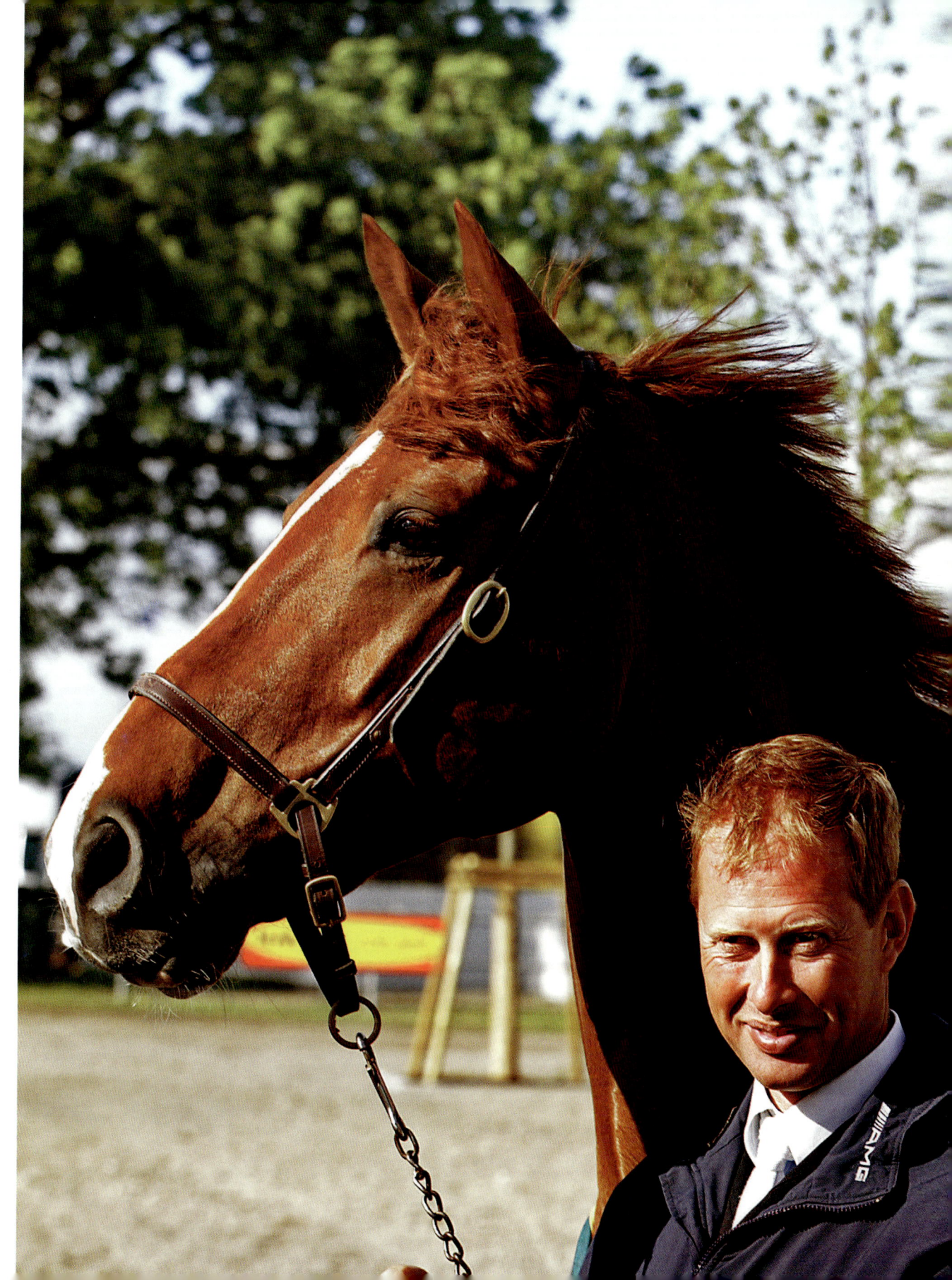

SPORT HORSE SOUNDNESS AND PERFORMANCE

Let the horse advance step by step

Libero H: World Cup Champion 1994, set several records in the World Cup. Later, he was a successful sire (Jos Lansink)

Libero H was six years old when he and Jos started doing 1.20m classes at shows organised by the Dutch Rural Riders Association.

'He did not have much experience and it did not feel then that he would be a star. He was a "baby" when he came to us. It was a question of developing him, at home through training and then at shows, step by step. When it felt as though he could do more we brought him to the next level. When he had done something good he was rewarded by coming down a notch again. It was clear from early on that he needed the right management. You could not do a big class every day. At that age you should not ask too much anyway', said Jos, who at the time was stable jockey for Hans Horn.

The onlookers at shows were not kind: 'When he did 1.20m people said he would not make it at 1.30m and when he was doing 1.30m people said he would not be good enough at 1.40m. I will never forget the first time he did a 1.40m and had the first fence down and people said, "You see, his limit is 1.30m!"', Jos said with an amused tone.

Cento: Olympic team gold 2000, World Cup Champion 2001, later also a successful sire (Otto Becker)

When Otto Becker got Cento he was doing 1.20–1.30m classes. Cento was by nature careful over fences, and sensitive. Otto felt that he had to give him time, and did so. If he had done some big classes one weekend he was dropped down a level the next show. Cento could jump so big that he scared himself, and therefore it was better to wait while he was building his own confidence, Otto explained. He was also careful about not pushing the stallion against the clock. Results fluctuated a bit when Cento was eight or nine, but with an upward trend.

'The first season he was really consistent was in 2000', Otto Becker said. Then they won the World Cup in 's-Hertogenbosch, the Grosser Preis von Aachen and team gold in Sydney.

Opposite: **Carl Hester with Nip Tuck were members of the UK's medal teams at the World Equestrian Games in 2014, the European Championships 2015 and the Olympics in 2016, plus bronze medallist in the 2017 World Cup Final. The horse is very sensitive and before he started competing internationally he was travelling along with other horses to shows with groom Alan Davies without competing, just to get used to the environment. (Photo: Roland Thunholm.)**

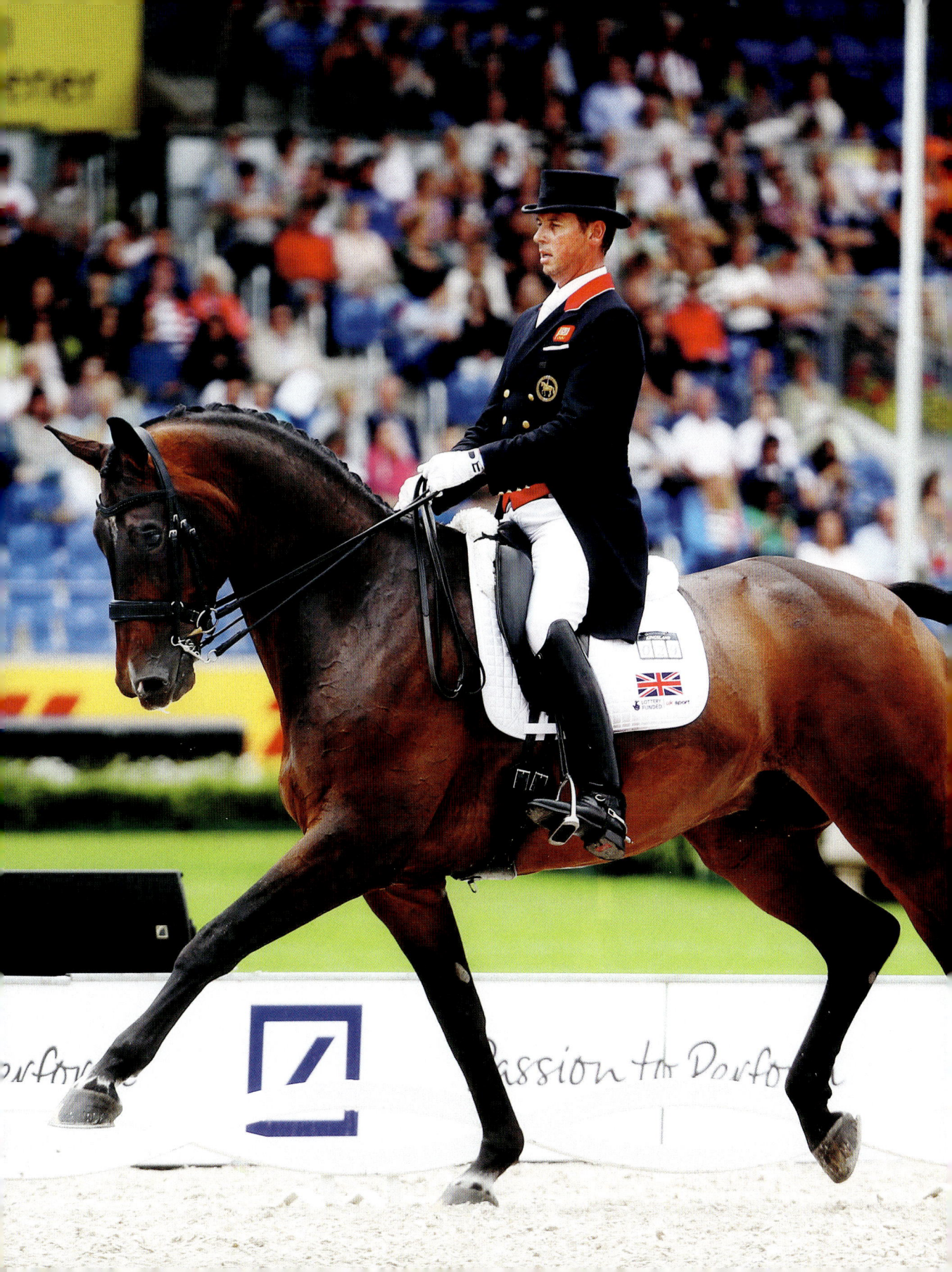

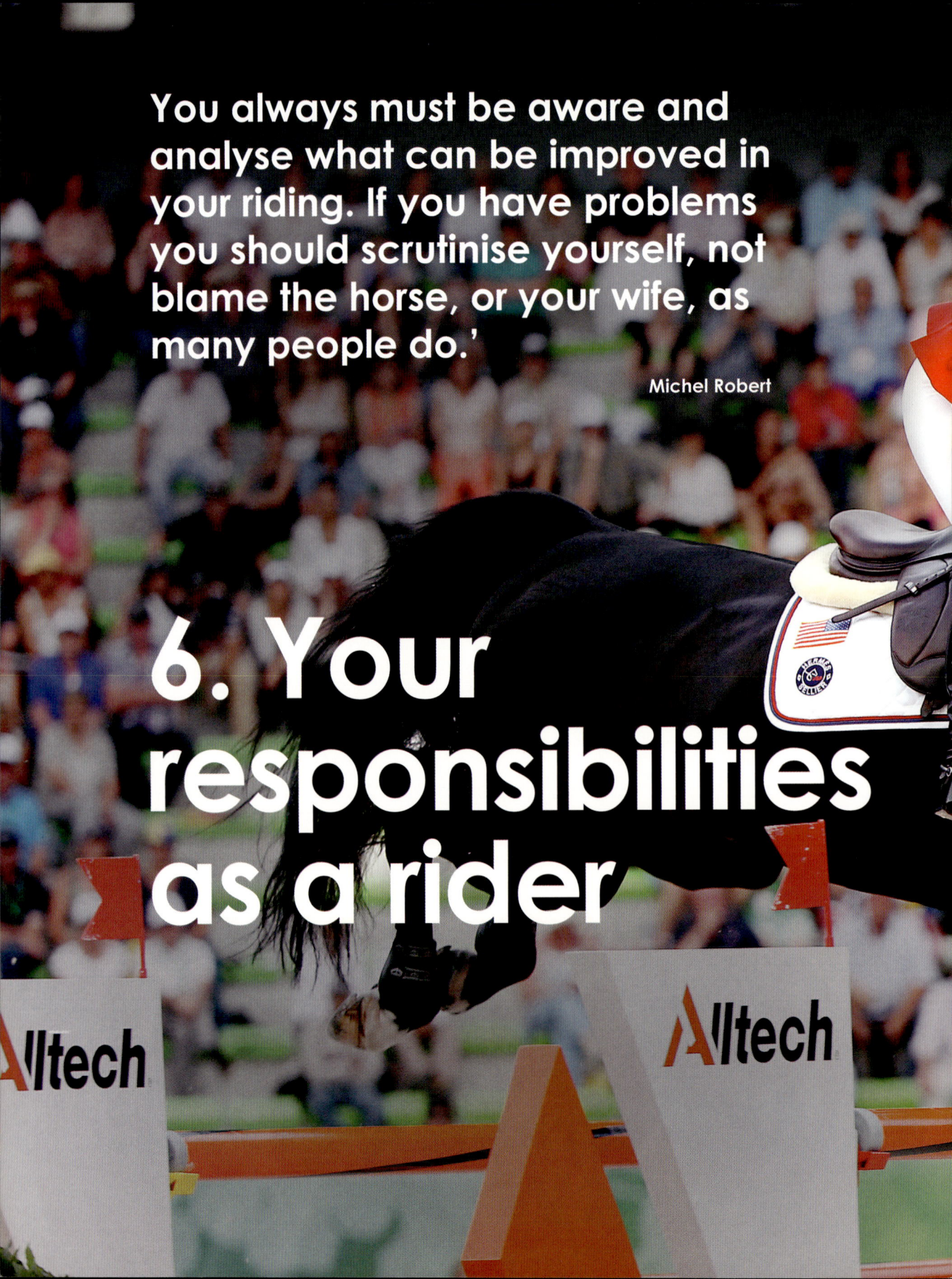

You always must be aware and analyse what can be improved in your riding. If you have problems you should scrutinise yourself, not blame the horse, or your wife, as many people do.'

Michel Robert

6. Your responsibilities as a rider

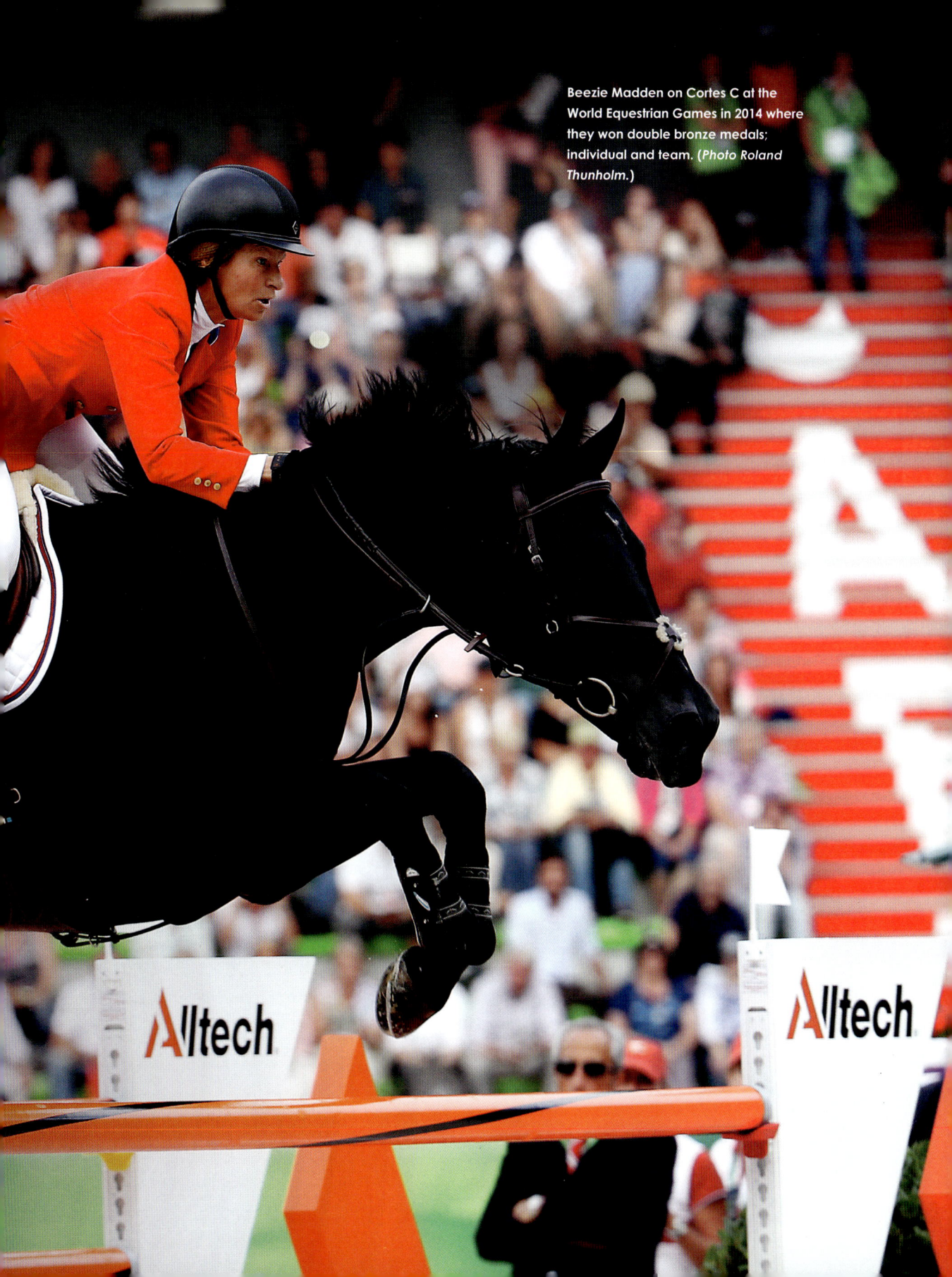

Beezie Madden on Cortes C at the World Equestrian Games in 2014 where they won double bronze medals; individual and team. (*Photo Roland Thunholm.*)

SPORT HORSE SOUNDNESS AND PERFORMANCE

THE HORSE'S MANAGER – YOU

From a distance it might be easy to think that champion riders in general are very sure of their own superiority. In fact, what they often have in common is a constant self-evaluation and striving to improve further, and not blaming the horse. One example is Peder Fredricson, double Olympic silver medallist who, since a young age, has been identified as a huge natural talent. 'All riders want to get better. If you don't have that drive to think about and work on how you can develop yourself you will never get really good', Peder said.

Who trains and 'shapes' the horse? You as a rider! both Peder and Franke Sloothaak said this. This, of course, means that you must pay a lot of attention to your own training and development, in order to be able to help the horse in the best way possible. Other top names have the same view.

'The rider must reflect about everything, and have a broad view', Franke said. It includes feeding, training and rest. The rider should also pay constant attention to how the horse feels and functions, and if something does not feel right. On this issue, Franke had the following advice:

'If you have a problem you must address it and try to solve it. Not doing that is probably a key weakness in some riders. They hope that it will solve itself tomorrow. But if you do nothing it will not get better. If something with the horse is not as it should be, you must be able to spot that, analyse possible reasons and what can be done. Is the horse maybe in pain? You must always try to understand how every horse functions, what he feels, what he needs. You can never do too much of that.'

YOUR RESPONSIBILITIES AS A RIDER

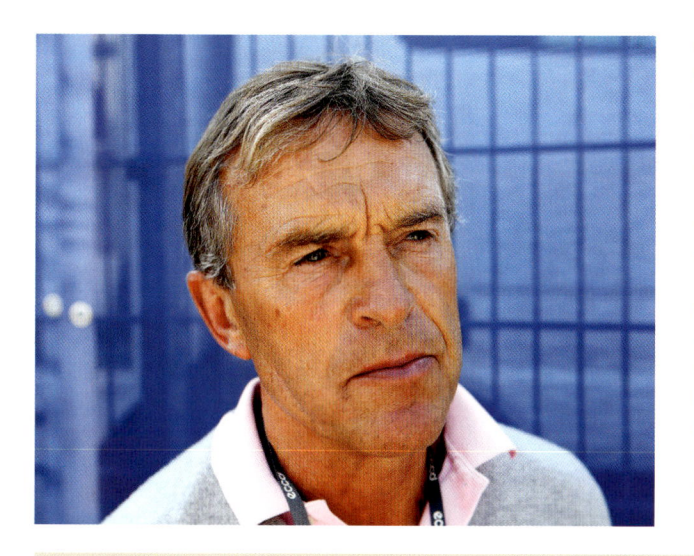

Henk Nooren was formerly one of Holland's best team riders, including being close to a place in the final four at the 1978 World Championships. He has since become one of the world's most successful coaches and chefs d'equipe. Henk was the team coach when Sweden broke an eighty-year medal drought to win a triple of team silvers at the 2001 Europeans, 2002 World Equestrian Games and 2004 Olympics, and again when Rolf Göran Bengtsson was European Champion in 2011 and when the team won European bronze in 2013. He has also been in charge of the French, Spanish and Italian national teams. (*Photo Roland Thunholm.*)

Top coach Henk Nooren: attention to detail and 'helicopter view'

One of the strengths and secrets of top showjumping coach Henk Nooren is being able to analyse and understand each horse down to the minutest detail, according to Swedish team rider Malin Baryard-Johnsson.

' Nothing, nothing at all must be left to chance', he said straight after Sweden won Olympic team silver at Athens in 2004. 'It can be a question of rideability, of a niggling injury, how the horse is shod. There are masses of details that can make a difference. '

Henk has seldom gone home from an international championship without 'his' team winning a medal. One example of his attention to detail was during the Swedish team's pre-camp ahead of the 2004 Olympics: 'Every day I went through every team horse probably twenty-five times, until I was completely fed up with myself', he said afterwards. He then also analysed the competition schedule, which included evening jumping under floodlights. The Swedish horses got to practise under floodlights beforehand, as being unfamiliar with floodlights can spook a horse. The team also practised different types of water features and types of fences that could be expected to be included in the Olympic courses.

'After the last training session on the final day before going to Athens we could not know if we would get a medal, but we did know that all horses were at peak fitness', Henk said.

All horses have some weakness, whether imperfect technique or something else. It is the rider's job to help the horse overcome that. But – and this is key – many problems in riding and with the horse are actually down to the rider, in the experience of both top riders and vets. Eventing star Pippa Funnell said in an interview that about 85 per cent of problems with the horse are caused by the rider. In 2014 Pippa's and her showjumping European gold medallist husband William's students included three of Europe's most prominent young riders; Anna Wilks who won the Junior Europeans in eventing, Sweden's Hedwig Wik, who was seventh in the Young Rider Europeans in eventing and their former stable jockey Spencer Roe, who was on the UK showjumping team at the World Equestrian Games at the age of just twenty-one. One of Pippa's cornerstones with a new student is to go back to basics, work on establishing correct foundations and giving that process enough time.

That is also a key message from French jumping legend Michel Robert: 'You must have a correct seat, that is very, very important. If you have the right seat and the right attitude everything else will be easy. But it is difficult to sit correctly on the horse; you might be too stiff, you might be crooked in a shoulder or a knee. All that will be felt by the horse.'

IMPROVING YOURSELF MENTALLY AND PHYSICALLY

Many champions and other top riders make a point of going back to basics, getting help to look at their weaknesses or what can be improved, and working on that. It again comes back to attention to detail. Real riding skill is a lot about timing, co-ordination and feel, which do require time in the saddle to develop. Not everyone has the chance, determination or resources to get maximum time in the saddle, to ride full-time, or even as much as they would like. But there are many

YOUR RESPONSIBILITIES AS A RIDER

aspects to success in riding that you can improve off the horse, that top riders pay attention to.

Reflect about your own profile as a rider concerning:

- Modesty and self-confidence.
- Balance and body control/awareness.
- Physical strength, fitness and suppleness.
- Your weight and what you eat (too much, too little or just right?).
- Mental attitude and sports psychology.
- Your knowledge about horses and their care, and what team of experts you have around the horse.

You can develop all these aspects, and then also improve your and your horse's chances to succeed.

Modesty and self-confidence (have someone's eyes on the ground!)

Champion riders often point out how important the rider's mental attitude is in performance. Modesty is then a key factor. It is about being humble towards the horse, about your own riding, and to what extent you are prepared to try to improve and work towards your goals. At the same time most successful riders have a portion of self-confidence or self-belief, and perseverance. When Franke Sloothaak listed the factors necessary to succeed in riding the first point was: 'You can do it if you want it, everything is possible if you really want it.' He went on:

'But some never get started, they give up straight away. There are riders who have more talent than I have. But maybe they don't use their head enough, or do not work hard enough. To succeed you need several factors; you must have some talent, find horses and be at the right place at the right time. It is a question of personality as well, are you prepared to work hard?

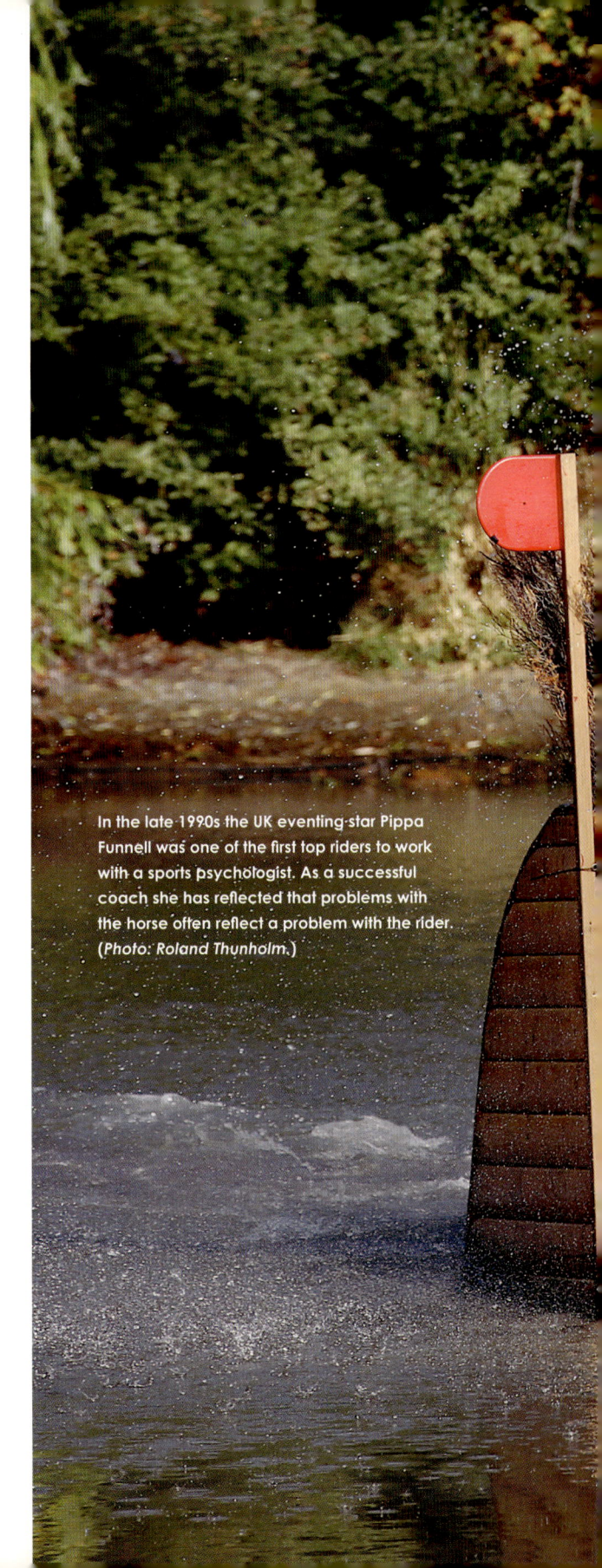

SPORT HORSE SOUNDNESS AND PERFORMANCE

There are those with talent, who do not want to do the work or are not intelligent enough. There are those who are intelligent enough but do not have the talent – everything must fit. But you can say the same about riders as with horses, if someone has one weakness it can be compensated by something else. You never get to the point that you are the best at everything.'

The very best riders always look at how they can improve further. Michel Robert explained in an interview what he meant when talking about trying to make progress every day. He had, after all, already been at the top level for more than forty years. His reply was chosen as the key quote for this chapter: 'OK, I can ride, but you always have to pay attention to, and analyse, what you can do better as a rider. If you have a problem in riding you should look at yourself, not blame the horse, or your wife, as many people do.'

When asked what changes he has made in trying to improve, Robert replied that he has become stronger mentally.

'Do not blame the horse if something does not work', is also a comment from Michael Whitaker, who also has some forty years in the sport. He went on: 'All horses can't reach top level, but you should be able to find a system that suits that particular horse, and help him to become as good as he can with the level of talent he has.'

In the late 1990s the UK eventing star Pippa Funnell was one of the first top riders to work with a sports psychologist. As a successful coach she has reflected that problems with the horse often reflect a problem with the rider. (Photo: Roland Thunholm.)

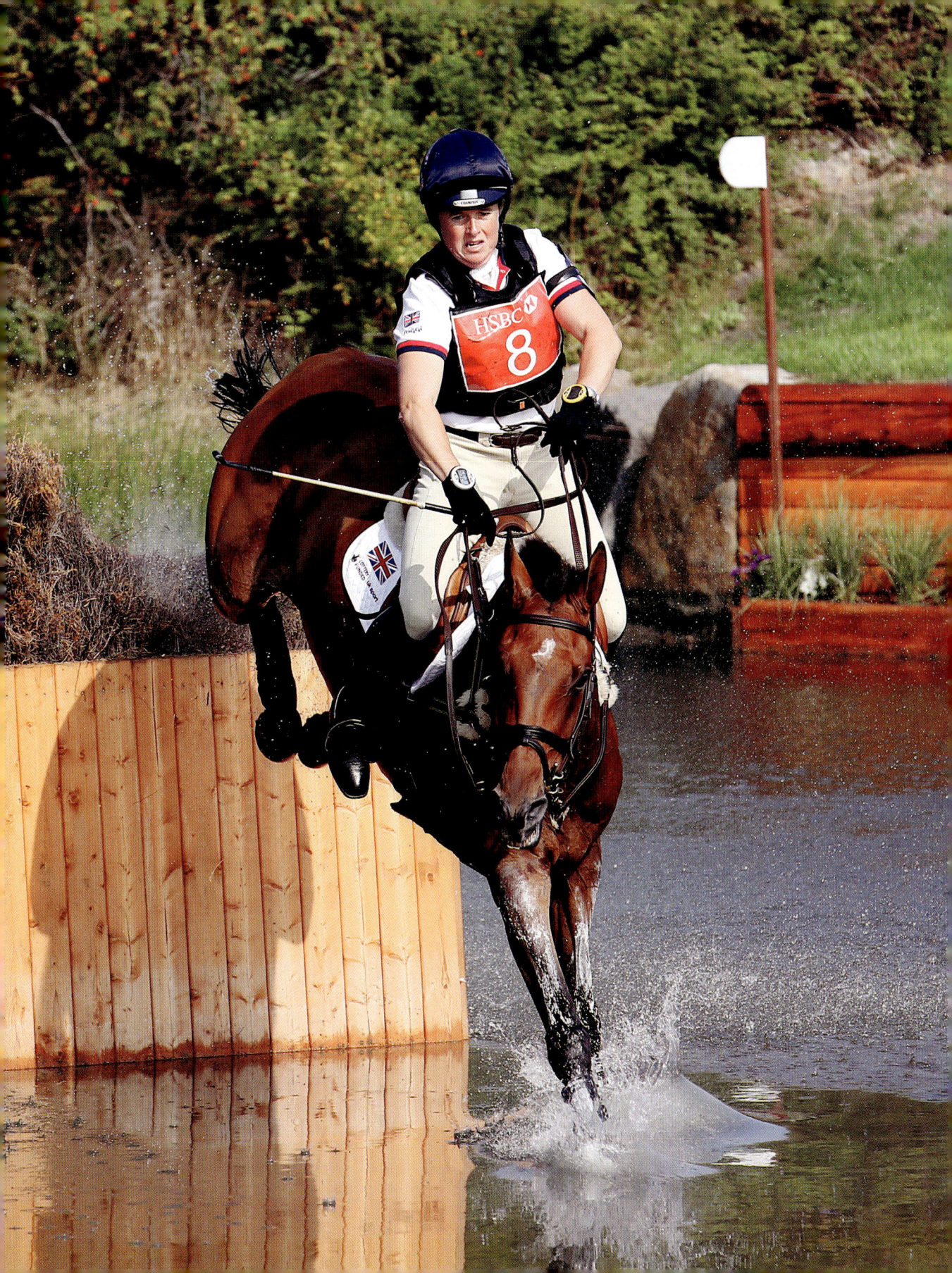

European bronze medallist Jens Fredricson has used similar wording; 'Horsemanship is to help the horse to realise his potential at whatever level.'

The attitude of these riders is that you can always improve and you can always learn from someone else, including in disciplines other than your own.

Eventing legend Sir Mark Todd has been getting dressage coaching from Charlotte Dujardin. When Sir Mark won his first Olympic gold in eventing in 1984 Charlotte was not even born, but of course since then she has won ten gold medals in dressage.

Rodrigo Pessoa was just twenty-plus and hailed as a riding wunderkind when he decided to become a dressage student of the famous rider and coach Georg Theodorescu and his daughter Monica (later Germany's dressage chef d'equipe). Rodrigo's father, Nelson, also had dressage training in his younger days, with the then-leading German rider Willy Schultheiss, and used what he learnt in developing the flatwork of his showjumpers.

When Dutch dressage icon Anky van Grunsven was experiencing problems with steady halts she took advice from the Dutch reining champion – and started competing in reining herself, winning a bronze medal in the 2015 Europeans.

When Ludger Beerbaum was in his early twenties and had won a Young Rider European Championship medal and started working for Paul Schockemöhle, he rode some ten horses a day. He then he stayed on after his own work and watched and carried poles for his more senior colleague Franke Sloothaak, to watch him train.

On balance, seat and body control

Michel Robert

'The rider must understand how he influences the horse with his seat, as this is very important for the horse. Many riders have a need to learn more about how the horse functions physically and mentally, and about how they influence the horse. If the rider has a good seat and the horse is in a good physical shape, dressage or flatwork is simple. But if you sit incorrectly on a horse in poor physical shape it is difficult. When I am training a student I do a lot of work on the seat. It is very important that the rider has someone on the ground to help with that, because it is very, very difficult to correct yourself. You must work on your seat every day. You need to be aware what is your own specific problem; only then you will be able to work on it, a little bit at a time. The right seat and style of riding is not something you learn from one single person. I am still working on my own seat every day.'

Franke Sloothaak

'Almost all problems that occur with the horse are down to lack of balance, either in the rider or the horse. If the rider is in balance, the horse will be in balance. If the horse is running away after a fence it is because of lack of balance, that the rider is too far forward with his upper body', Franke said. He underlined that balance and training the seat are closely related, and that the seat is also very important in flatwork.

When eventing champion Pippa Funnell talked about the fact that 85 per cent of problems in the horse can be down to the rider, her point is supported by experienced sport horse vets. They regularly come across horses who the rider finds a challenge to ride, or that seem to have a mild lameness. The rider suspects a physical problem. But when, as part of the clinical investigation, a more experienced rider gets up instead, the problem disappears straight away. What have been interpreted as lamenesses or resistances are in fact the consequences of poor riding or poor communication with the horse.

Sport horse vets and physiotherapists who work with both riders and horses have made the observation that physical problems in the rider can cause problems in the horse. Among examples were:

1. Rider hip/back problems.
2. Poor rider balance (compare this with John Whitaker's last bullet point in Chapter 3).
3. Uneven hands.

When the rider receives treatment and recovers the horse recovers, based on their experiences.

SPORT HORSE SOUNDNESS AND PERFORMANCE

Meeting the researcher

'It is not enough trying to improve your balance if you don't know why you have poor balance.' – Maria Terese Engell.

Everyone talks about the fact that the horse should be straight in his body, but is the rider himself straight or crooked? Equine vet and biomechanical researcher Maria Terese Engell from Norway has a background as both dressage rider and ballet dancer. From childhood she observed her father Håvard's work on co-ordination, balance and movement with Norway's top athletes in different disciplines, on behalf of the Norwegian Olympic Committee. She initiated a scientific research project into rider body posture and balance with the help of the equine biomechanics groups at the Swedish University of Agricultural Sciences, and received funding from the double Olympic dressage medallist Ulla Håkansson.

In Maria Terese's research high-speed cameras and sensors are used to capture rider movement not visible to the eye.

For optimal performance – and the horse's well-being – riders should not only have a correct and balanced posture but also move the body parts independently and appropriately to be synchronised with and absorb the horse's motion.

'A horse can feel and will react to a fly on his body. Imagine then what he feels from the rider', Maria Terese said.

To learn to ride is, to an important extent, to develop one's ability to be able to synchronise with and absorb the movement of the horse, and the higher the level of equestrian sport the more important this becomes, Maria Terese points out. For good performance a rider is dependent on good body control, balance and rhythm, and this is being analysed in her research.

'In all sports you come back to co-ordination and balance and figuratively break down the individual movements into parts, a bit like building blocks, until you spot where the fundamental weakness is. Then you work on the different parts, and put them back together', Maria Terese says.

'The horse will move in the best possible way only if he is not restricted by the rider being out of balance or asymmetrical in his own body. Riding is, in essence, a communication between horse and rider. For the communication to work the aids must be correct and precise in relation to the horse's movement. This is only possible if the rider has been able to develop a good body control and body awareness', Maria Terese points out. A lot of riders unconsciously give contradictory signals to the horse through lack of balance and asymmetrical body patterns. Have you had or seen a lesson where the riding teacher/coach tells you/the student to correct something, and you/the student protest(s) and is convinced you/they are doing something else?

If and when a horse is subject to contradictory signals and demands this can result in injury, in Maria Terese's and other equine vets' experience.

When working with riders Maria Terese and her father do not offer any 'quick-fix' seat solutions, but work on finding the individual imbalances followed by a gradual process (including daily homework) with slow exercises designed to establish new postural habits and to 're-programme' the brain and body.

All riders need to be strong and solid in their trunk, or core. A jumping rider needs at the same time to have strength and to be supple, and a dressage rider needs to have a naturally strong posture and body control to absorb the power from the horse. The rider who has not, for example, developed a correct back posture and is using the wrong muscles to keep himself upright, will be stiff and bounce in the saddle', Maria Terese said.

Seat training

Training the seat and a correct balance are very important factors in the systems of many top coaches. Students at the Spanish Riding School in Vienna spend their first whole year only being lunged, to establish a correct seat. The same principle was valid at the famous training centre Waterstock in England, run by Lars Sederholm. There, already successful riders were also lunged to work on their seat. It can be difficult to get access to private seat training with a coach, but there is increasing research about rider body control and balance.

Physical strength, suppleness and fitness

There have been many changes in international top-level showjumping in the past fifteen or twenty years. One of them is that the top riders have started working on their own fitness and strength. Rolf Göran Bengtsson noted in an interview that he and other top riders in the past focused solely on their horses' fitness and did not set aside time for their own. Elite showjumping riders have more injuries than many onlookers realise, but one aspect of fitness training is that it can help prevent this. Incidentally, one study of Swedish event riders showed that they suffered more 'overuse' injuries than accidents.

When top riders talk of their own physical training they mean both cardio and strength training, as in running or in the gym, as well as suppleness and core strength training as in Pilates and yoga.

Henrik von Eckermann's long-term boss Ludger Beerbaum has been a pioneer of the trend of improved rider fitness. When working for Ludger, Henrik trained four or five days a week. He ran, did strength training and balance work. The Beerbaum stable had its own personal trainer who came once a week to work with the riders. Henrik added: 'The show hotels often have a gym. Early in the morning you always meet one or several of the other riders there. Fifteen years ago they would all still have been asleep in bed.'

Beezie Madden has told of starting to go to a gym a few years ago and finding it beneficial in her riding.

The Swedish Olympic Committee's personal trainer Jesper Sjökvist works with Swedish team riders and has a wide experience of other sports. He points out that, if the rider is fit and strong, the horse's job gets easier. 'If you have good body strength you can keep your position in the saddle better. Horse and rider should be as one, and then the rider must be able to keep his own position so that the horse does not have to compensate for the rider's lack of balance', he said.

Jesper strongly rebuts the non-equestrian cliché that 'riders are not athletes, it is the horse who does the work'. His experience is that no athletes work harder than top riders! His reflection is also that they are athletic with good co-ordination and suppleness, but when some top riders are not in peak fitness it is precisely because they work so hard and ride so many horses daily that they have little time for their own training.

Jesper is in charge of the physical/personal training project for elite and talent groups that the Olympic Committee started in 2013, for eventers, dressage riders and jumping riders. He is a former weightlifter who has worked with physical training in half a dozen ball sports. In addition he has worked with US university team athletes in track and field, tennis, gymnastics, swimming, cross-country running, boxing and sailing.

Jesper's work includes helping riders to plan physical training programmes for themselves and, at the same time, test their strength, suppleness and endurance. Those results he then uses to analyse what is the right 'physical profile' for each sport and discipline. Training aimed at preventing injury is included.

Swedish team rider Douglas Lindelöw follows a personal

trainer programme he was given by Jesper with for example, push-ups and sit-ups. One focus for him has been improved core strength. In addition Douglas goes running, about 4–5km per session. Both he and World Equestrian Games semi-finalist Alexander Zetterman believe that it gives a competitive edge to be well-trained physically.

'I think you have an advantage against other competitors if you can keep your focus and have more strength. If you are fit, everything else is much easier. You feel more alert, with more energy. You also get more supple and soft in your body when riding, and more able to move in harmony with your horse', Alexander said. He does physical exercise almost daily, or every other day, fitness and strength training. Alexander has some equipment at home, for example a spinning bike and machines, but likes also to go to a gym in order to focus on the training.

Your weight and what you eat

Many riders pay enormous attention to what their horse eats, but forget about their own nutrition. As with physical training this is something that seems to be changing at elite level. Beezie Madden has noted that it can be very difficult not to eat junk food when out at shows. She and her husband John got advice from their personal trainer to put together guidelines. 'We try to plan our meals and eat healthily with mainly low-fat protein, whole grains and fruit and vegetables', she said.

Jesper Sjöqvist said that the Swedish Olympic Committee have started working with team riders on nutrition, to help them eat sensibly and promote their focus and energy levels: 'It is a priority area where we get help from nutritional experts. They help the riders to find a strategy in their everyday life including a time schedule, so that they do, for example, eat lunch, instead of grabbing half a sandwich and then feel ravenous later, and they have planned light, healthy snacks between meals. Skipping lunch does not work in the long run; you lose your concentration.'

Other riders are heavier than they should be. How much weight a horse can carry can be a sensitive question. Not a lot of scientific tests have been done, but both one with horses working on a treadmill and cavalry handbooks of old suggest that a horse should not carry more than 20 per cent of his own weight. For a 500kg horse this means 100kg for the rider and saddle together. The build of the horse is also a factor, based on the same treadmill study and traditional experience.

Jesper Sjökvist's PT programme for jumping riders

We try to demonstrate to the riders that you can do training sessions at home and even in the stable, without having to go to a gym. You can put together a programme of about 30 minutes. The most important point is that it actually gets done, regularly. In Sweden, post-hole augers have been used for weight training; some people have bought dumbbells. With a bit of imagination you can manage. Again, you can do several of these exercises in the stable.

Kneebends while lifting a weight such as described.
Jesper: 'Develops both core body strength and mobility in the hips.'

Lunges.
Jesper: 'Good exercise for riders, who often are stiff in their hips. We want them to open up at the hip and get stronger there.'

Push-ups.

Chin-ups.
Jesper: 'If possible it is good to have a bar set up in a door and practise lifting yourself by the arms.'

Sit-ups etc.

Running.
Jesper: 'You can run almost anywhere and anytime.'

A horse with more bone and a wider back has better weight-carrying capacity than a lighter-built animal.

Mental attitude and sports psychology

Mental training has become a focus among top riders in the past ten to twenty years. Quite a few consult their own mental coach, and some federations and Olympic Committees have sports psychology as part of their team programmes. Sweden's former team coach Henk Nooren found mental attitude in the riders so important that he himself studied the subject at university level.

Many riders do not have the funds or opportunity to consult a private sports psychologist, but there is plenty of material on mental training to study, through books, DVDs and web-based talks.

When Sweden's Peder Fredricson set an Olympic record with six rounds without fences down at Rio and won individual Olympic silver, mental training had been an important part of his preparations. All his connections noticed his focus. He had been working with sports psychologists from the Swedish Olympic Committee, but in the run-up to Rio also studied books he bought on the internet about the mental training of the US Navy SEALS elite forces. The idea in several of the books written about and by Navy SEALS is that the mental strength they need in a military operation also gives an advantage to others faced with challenging situations.

'It was almost a bit scary when I asked "How would you feel now if you got nervous or stressed?" and he just replied "That's not going to happen". He is so bloody focused', his wife Lisen (herself a two-time Olympic rider) said in a TV documentary. About a week later Peder and H&M All In were second to Nick Skelton and Big Star in a six-horse jump-off. 'I knew that I had a very good horse and that if I didn't make any mistakes I had the chance of a medal and even gold', Peder said about riding H&M All In and his preparations for Rio.

So why mental training for Peder, who had already won an Olympic team silver in 2004? Sylve Söderstrand was the Swedish chef d'equipe at that time, and the coach at Rio.

'Peder is an amazing rider, who thinks like a horse and almost is like a horse', Sylve said, 'but at important shows he sometimes has been given instructions that he could not process and use on the course.' This did not happen in Rio.

'Whatever you do, you should reflect about how you can do it better. It can be about feed, your own riding, etc., apart from how you function mentally', Peder said. 'Mental training is not only about not getting nervous, but a whole package; to move forward, improve yourself. Mental training is personal development, not just about nerves but how you prioritise.'

(Eventing champion Pippa Funnell described the same analysis of the rider's situation as a whole when she consulted a sports psychology coach in the late 1990s.)

Among the important techniques Peder learnt was developing an 'on and off' button. This means being able to switch on and focus completely when you are expected to perform, and then relax fully in between. This is useful at the Olympics, where there is a lot of waiting time.

Another technique Peder used was not thinking 'if'. This is the same principle that Pippa Funnell learnt when working to get out of a pattern when she was in the lead after the dressage, but got nervous ahead of the cross-country.

'You must follow your instinct; if you are governed by emotions you get weak. You must not be full of hope or worry, but be neutral', Peder said. 'You should not keep thinking about what happened or what might happen. You should just be in the "now", and not think about whether it is going well or badly. You also should not try to change something in the last minute, or think about what the other riders are doing, but focus on your own horse at that moment and on the course right then.'

SPORT HORSE SOUNDNESS AND PERFORMANCE

Mental attitude – don't give up, try again

The importance of not giving up after a setback but trying again is an important lesson in sports psychology. Two Olympic gold medallists from the past thirty years demonstrate that; Pierre Durand and Rodrigo Pessoa.

Rodrigo Pessoa

At the 2004 Athens Olympics Rodrigo considered not going in the last individual round. He was lying in twenty-third place. He ended the day as gold medallist, even if he did not get to receive it right then. Rodrigo and Baloubet du Rouet had won three World Cup Finals in a row, indoors. But in outdoor championships they had had a jinx. At the Sydney Olympics in 2000 Baloubet was eliminated for refusals, three fences from the finishing line and a gold medal. At the World Equestrian Games in 2002 Baloubet was eliminated again. Rodrigo decided not to do any more championships with the stallion, but changed his mind and went to Athens. There he had two fences down in the first round of the individual final and could not understand why, and was ready to give up and not start in the last round.

'I said that this is s**t. We have worked so hard and have had such great expectations, but it is pointless to continue', Rodrigo remembers. He was sitting in the stables during the interval with the Pessoa stable's coach Jos Klumps. Because of his low placing Rodrigo wanted to pull out of the second round. Klumps had trained Rodrigo from when he was a boy and calmed him down.

When they walked the course for the second round Rodrigo understood that his sense of failure had been premature, and that it was fortunate that Klumps had reassured him. Rodrigo's father, Nelson, said that when they started walking the second course they were rubbing their hands when seeing the fences, because the course was 'impossible'. And they knew this suited Baloubet, because there was never a fence that was too big or too difficult for him. Rodrigo was now clear, while those previously in the lead had fences down. Three horses went into the jump-off and Baloubet and Rodrigo won the silver – exchanged into gold when Cian O'Connor was later disqualified for a doping offence. (Sadly the third jump-off horse, Chris Kappler's Royal Kaliber, had a serious tendon injury on the course and later died from complications.)

YOUR RESPONSIBILITIES AS A RIDER

Pierre Durand

When Pierre Durand and the trotter cross Jappeloup won Olympic Gold in 1988 it was a complete contrast to four years earlier at the Los Angeles Olympics, and a further example of the importance of not giving up. At Los Angeles Jappeloup refused and Pierre fell off. That seemed to be the end of his Olympic dreams, which had started twenty years earlier when Pierre was thirteen years old and watching on television when French compatriot Pierre Jonqueres d'Oriola won the gold in Tokyo. When Durand first saw Jappeloup he did not look like the horse who would fulfil the Olympic dream, and after the refusals and falling off in LA it seemed unlikely. But Durand tried again and four years later won the individual gold in Seoul. In 2013 his and Jappeloup's story became the movie *Jappeloup*, which was very successful in France and is available as a DVD with English subtitles.

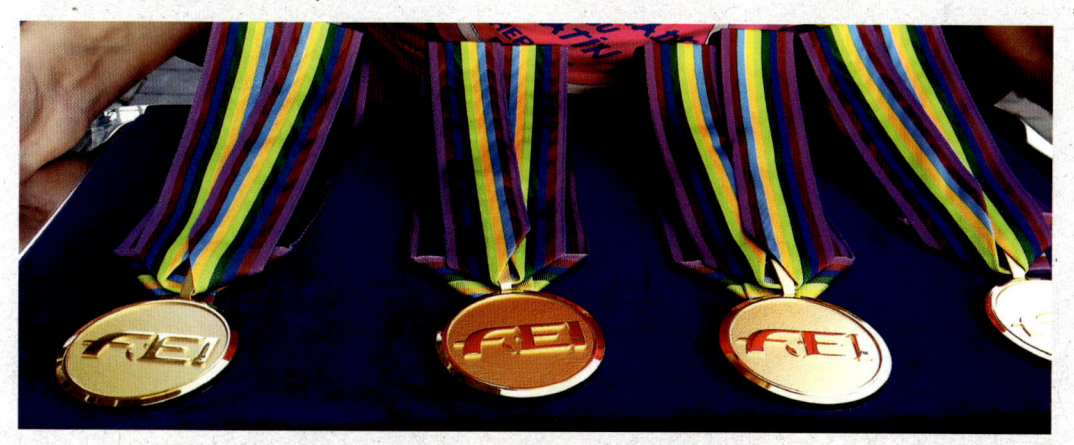

The team gold medals just before being presented to the winning Dutch team at the European Championships at Aachen in 2015. (*Photo: Dr Cecilia Lönnell.*)

Rodrigo and the map of Rome

One aspect of mental training is visualiation. When Rodrigo Pessoa, at only twenty-five years of age, prepared himself for the World Equestrian Games (World Championships) in Rome in 1998 he had a map of the city put up above his bed, so that it was the first thing he saw when he woke up and the last thing he saw before switching the lights off. He won the individual gold with Lianos.

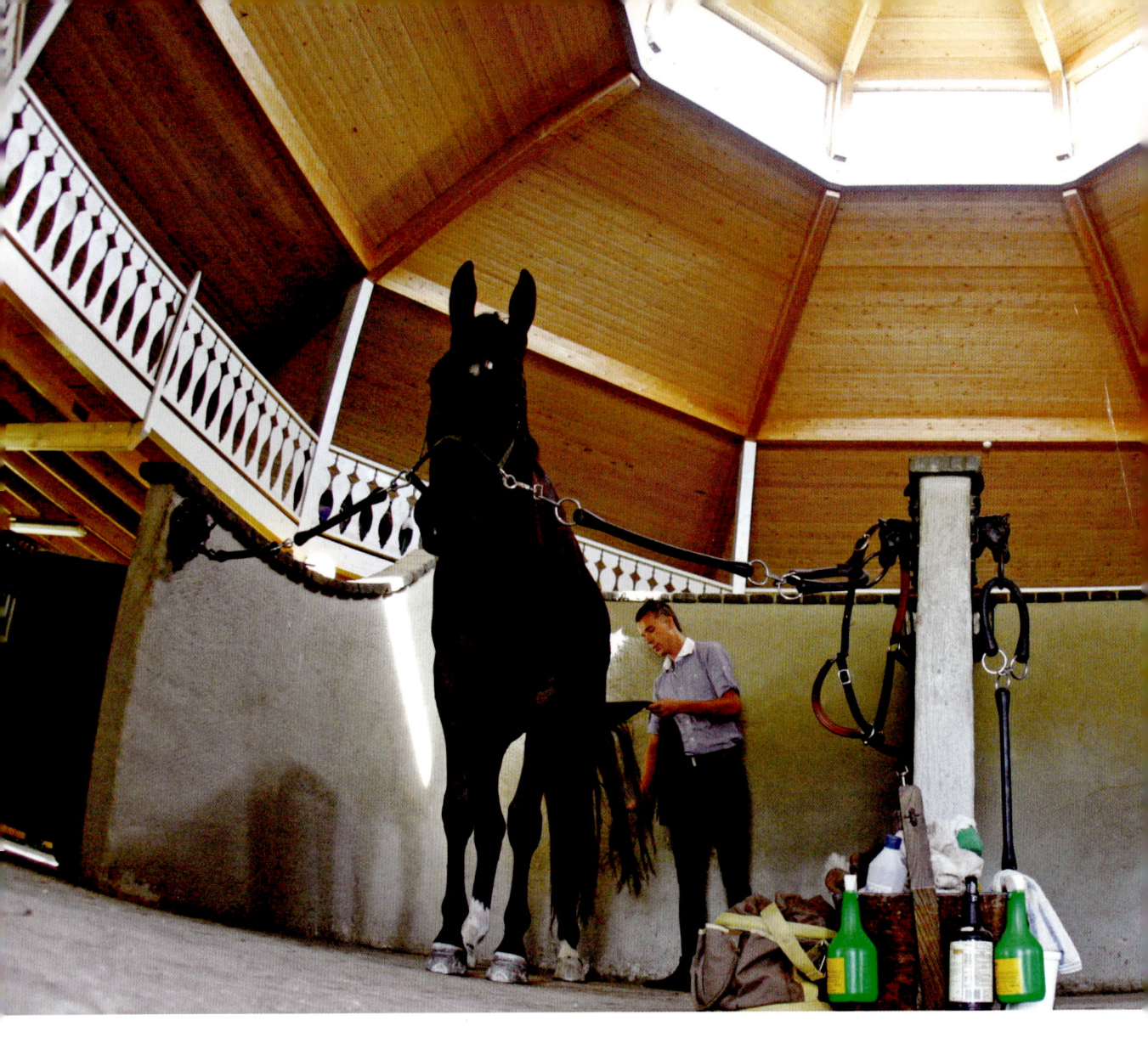

BUILD A SKILLED TEAM

Making a point of learning as much as possible about horse health and horse care is common advice from the experts. If you are not already involved in looking after horses, such as grooming, feeding or mucking out, make a point of it. The more time you spend with horses, the more you can learn about 'reading' them.

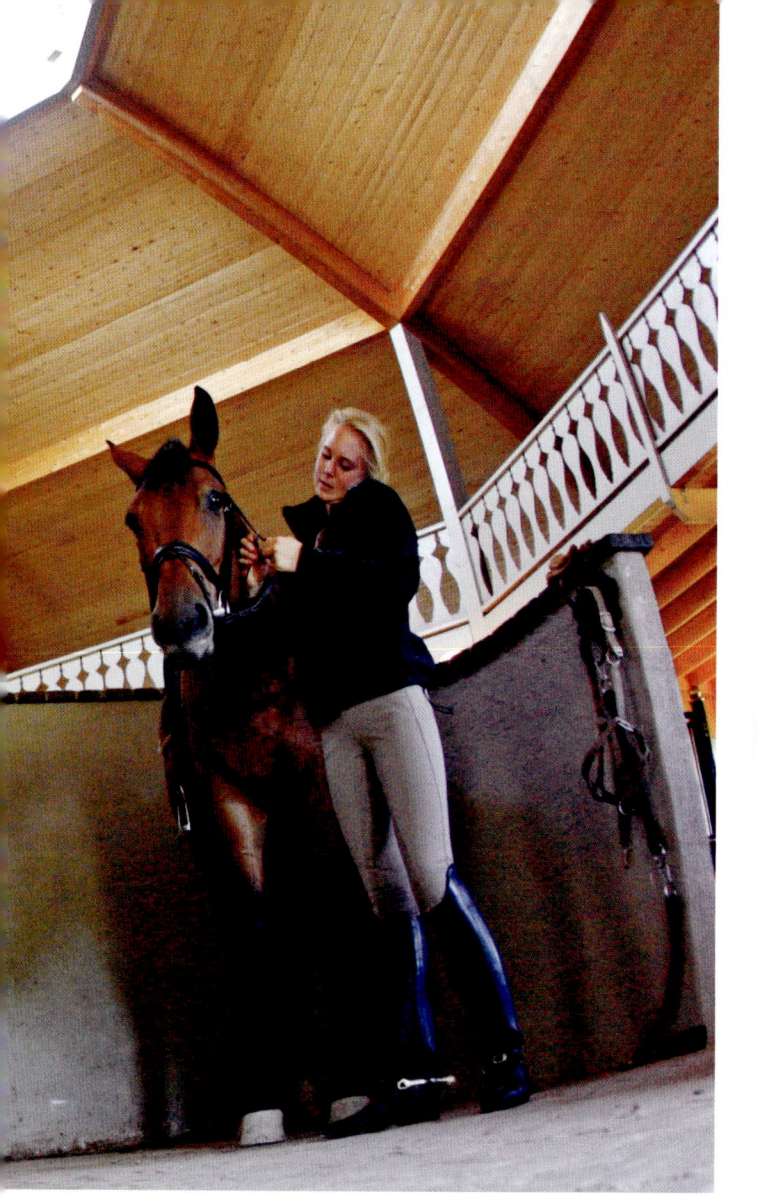

> **Reading suggestions**
>
> Most of the quotes by Michel Robert in this book are from an in-depth interview with the author carried out in Aachen some years back. But Robert has also described his philosophy and advice in his own book. One theme is the same as for this chapter, about the riders' attitude and way of thinking, especially in relation to the horse: Michel Robert **The Secrets and Method of a Great Champion**, Arthesis Communication 2005.

The whole care and management of the horse, including the stable environment, is important if he is to be able to feel good and perform. The dressage phenomenon Valegro (pictures elsewhere in the book) is groomed for an hour a day. His groom Alan Davies said that it has the effect of a light massage. (*Photo: Roland Thunholm.*)

Top riders in general also take advice from other specialists, and build a team of experts around the horse. In the champion riders' and vets' advice about preventing injury several point to the importance of the farrier – with expert trimming and shoeing. Several also mention the importance of working with an experienced equine vet. With a skilled team you are better positioned to prevent problems in the horse, or spot them early.

How to organise a health team and programme for your horse

1. If you are not already in regular contact with an experienced horse vet, do research on what equine clinics are available in your region, and/or find a specialist equine vet with an ambulatory practice. There are specialised equine vets and there are vets whose focus is more general large and/or small animal practice. An experienced equine vet is likely to have more in-depth skills regarding sport horses.
2. Ask your horse vet or other professionals who is the best farrier available. There are horse owners who bring their horse to an equine clinic with a resident farrier to get expert shoeing. In some countries there are lists available of farriers and their qualifications.
3. Get professional advice on analysing the stable environment, and on stable management. A horse who, for example, is subjected to poor air quality will not be able to perform, even if he is not lame.
4. Also get professional advice on checking your equipment and how it fits – certainly the saddle but also the bit, etc.
5. Ask your vet to teach you how to palpate your horse's legs and do that on a daily basis, so that you know what they should feel like when sound and healthy. You will then be able to detect signs of inflammation and injury, such as heat or swelling, as soon as they appear. Early discovery of, and response to, an injury will help in limiting the damage.
6. Find and cultivate a relationship with a skilled producer of hay or haylage. Do not try to save pennies on buying cheap feed, but pay for quality.
7. There are horse vets who work together with and can recommend, for example, equine physiotherapists, or complementary therapists, both for preventive treatments and for rehabilitation after an injury. For the horse's safety it is important not to bypass the vet, but have a clinical examination and diagnosis before any other treatments. (In the UK, it is a legal requirement to get a referral from a vet prior to treatment by these other therapists.)

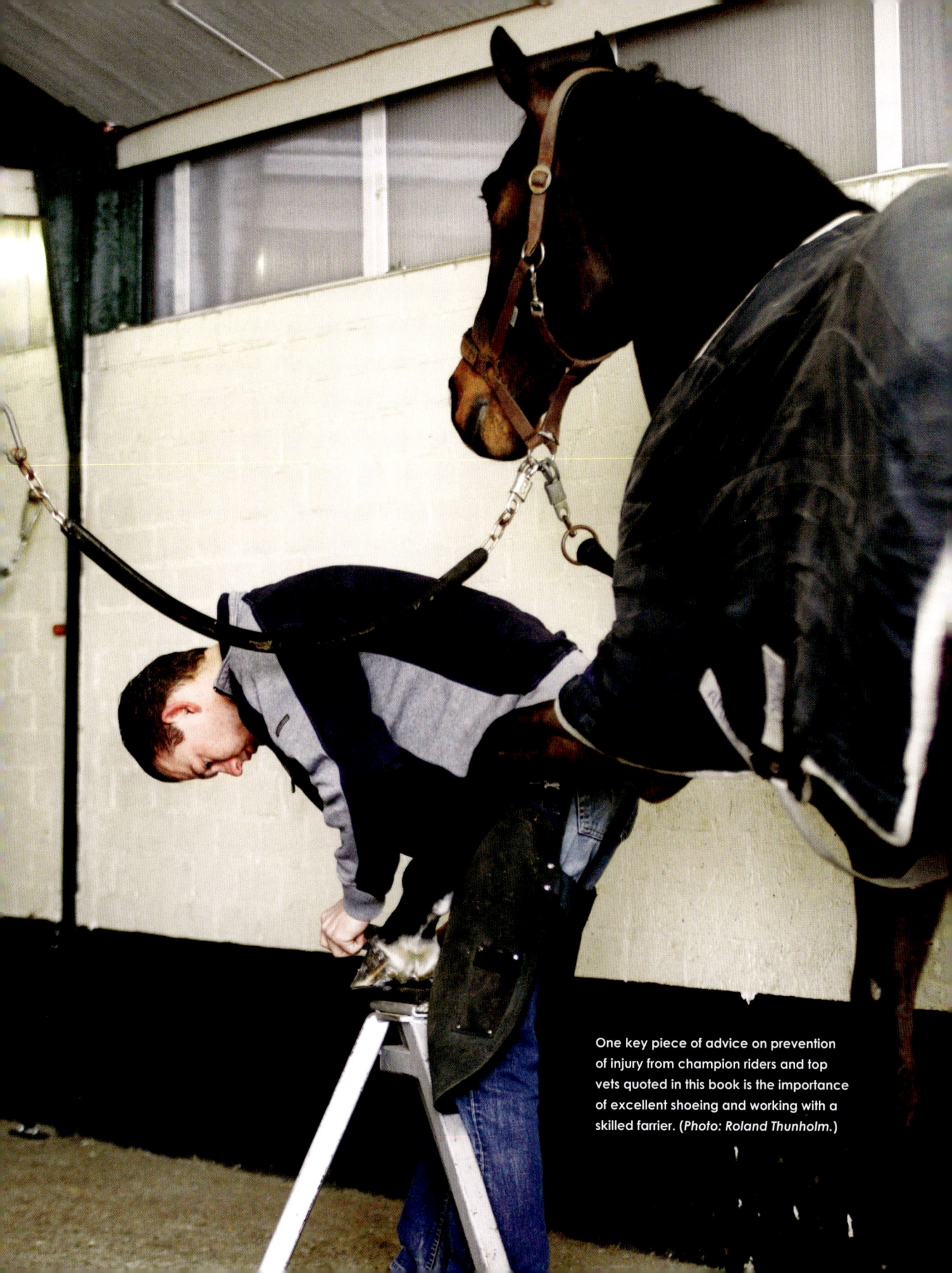

One key piece of advice on prevention of injury from champion riders and top vets quoted in this book is the importance of excellent shoeing and working with a skilled farrier. (*Photo: Roland Thunholm.*)

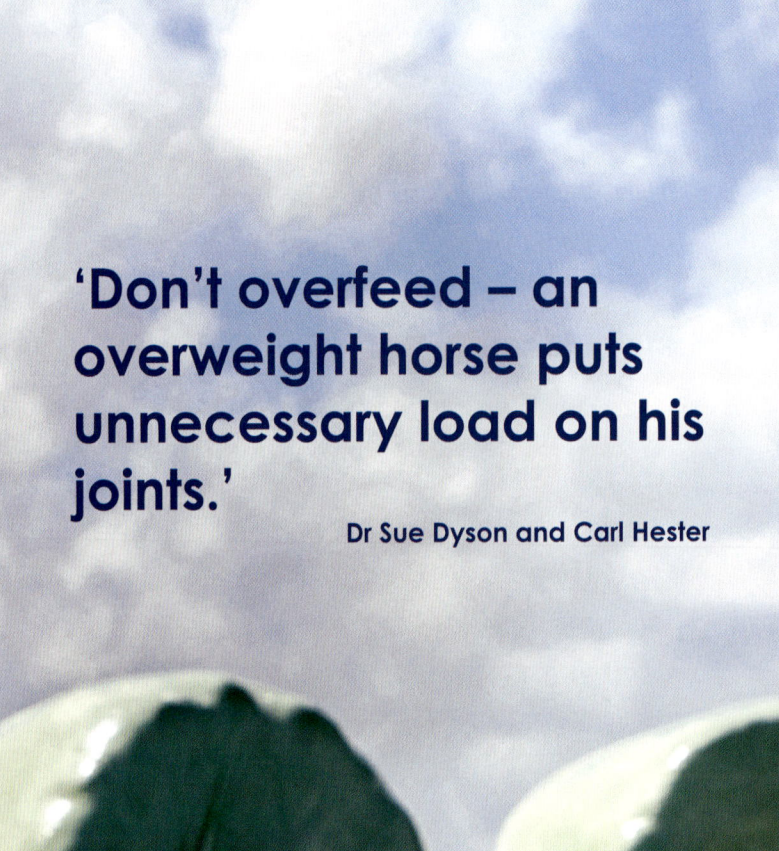

'Don't overfeed – an overweight horse puts unnecessary load on his joints.'

Dr Sue Dyson and Carl Hester

Photo: ThinkstockPhotos

7. Feeding, supplements and water

One aspect of performance and reading the horse is to give the right feed. It is the feed that provides fuel and building blocks for the body. Recent years have seen a shift in feeding strategies for top-level sport horses. The focus today is more towards a good-quality coarse feed, feeding several times a day and giving more fibre and less easily digested carbohydrates ('GI-diets'!). All this is more in tune with the horse's natural needs than giving plenty of hard feed and small/few portions of hay or haylage.

The EEHNC in Belgium in the spring of 2015 had feeding the sport horse as one of its key themes. The famous UK feed scientist and vet Dr Pat Harris gave a passionate talk about the importance of good-quality coarse feed for horses. She emphasised that the horse is, by nature, a grazing animal. The horse therefore has both a physical and mental need to eat grass (dried as in hay or haylage for storage purposes). In the wild it is natural for a horse to graze many hours per day, but he will consume a portion of hard feed in a few minutes. (Chapter 2 about the horse's body discusses these differences.)

Dr Pat Harris referred, for example, to a study from The Swedish University of Agricultural Sciences led by Professor Anna Jansson. It showed that young Standardbred trotters in training worked well on only haylage, provided it was an early harvest with high nutritional value.

In developed countries across the world it is nowadays more common for horses to be overfed rather than the other way around. Equine obesity has become an issue just as for humans and pets. Studies also show that some horse owners underestimate the horse's body score and do not spot signs of surplus weight.

'An overweight horse will put unnecessary load on his legs and joints, and run increased risk of metabolic syndrome', Dr Sue Dyson said in her soundness advice. She was referring to

'Buying new riding breeches? Please do, but first get a proper feed analysis'

This was the message in an advertisement for a Swedish feed laboratory a few years back, with World, European and Olympic medallist Peter Eriksson as the model. It might have been an advertisement, but is thought-provoking about the priorities of a rider or horse owner.

FEEDING, SUPPLEMENTS AND WATER

the realisation from scientific research that obese horses are at increased risk of developing laminitis.

Large portions of hard feed can result in the horse becoming overweight, and have also been shown to increase the risk of both colic and ulcers.

Poor feed hygiene is also suspected of increasing the risk of gastrointestinal disturbances and colic. Pay attention to choosing a really good-quality coarse feed, is the advice from Dr Sue Dyson. Her point fits in with Beezie Madden's advice:

1. Good hay should be the basis of the feeding (almost always a first crop for competition horses, as the hay made early in the season has higher nutritional value).
2. Give plenty of hay! Pay close attention to whether the hay has any signs of mould or similar, and discard that.
3. Before you spend lots of money on supplements, first make sure you do what is best for the horse regarding hay and hard feed.

The only supplement Beezie gives is a joint supplement, plus electrolytes when needed (that is in, hot weather or if the horse is otherwise sweating a lot). One important point made at the EEHNC was that, when horses are given electrolytes, it is very important that they also drink plenty of water.

Marketing supplements for horses is a massive industry, whereby many horse owners and riders spend vast amounts of money for products that, unlike the requirements for ordinary medicines, seldom have any proven effect. Anky van Grunsven commented in a panel discussion at the EEHNC that she was puzzled at the high number of different supplements some horse owners give their horses.

The thought that this or that product will keep the horse healthier or help him perform better can be tempting. But bear in mind this:

1. Either the product has no effect, and you have thrown away your money …
2. …or else they do have an effect and, in that case, you

> 'Good hay is the basis of our feeding regime … Before you spend a lot of money on supplements it is important to first be sure that you have done everything right for the horse regarding the fundamentals, roughage feed and hard feed.'
> Beezie Madden

Advice and warning!

Always read the contents label for feeds and supplements very carefully. Do not handle a product that does not display its contents. The International Equestrian Federation (FEI) website has a anti-doping section with specific warnings against supplements in particular.

SPORT HORSE SOUNDNESS AND PERFORMANCE

> **Reading suggestion**
>
> The feeding of the horse is a very important area to know about and understand as a rider. Apart from the health and performance aspects, the rider/horse owner can also become a more savvy consumer by learning more about feeding.
>
> *The Truth About Feeding Your Horse*, by Clare McLeod MSc RNutr (J.A. Allen/Crowood, 2007) is a comprehensive guide to all aspects of feeding, including for performance horse.

run the risk of breaking forbidden medication or doping rules! This is especially relevant for herbal products, that, for example, claim to have a calming effect.

Hard feed, for example oats, which contain plenty of starch (fast carbohydrates) can also affect the horse's behaviour. This is a traditional viewpoint that, in recent years, has been proved by studies.

One rider who reflected on this was Rodrigo Pessoa, with the Olympic and three-time World Cup Champion Baloubet du Rouet. One challenge with the stallion was harnessing his enormous natural energy, and the feeding was therefore something that the Pessoas analysed carefully. Baloubet did not get oats or barley, but a specially made muesli that, in combination with the roughage, covered his needs. One piece of the puzzle was that his daily lunch was a big serving of carrots, instead of ordinary feed – 'and then the right amount of work', Rodrigo said.

When you are determining the nutritional needs of your horse, do have a look at the heart rate table and levels of physical exertion that are discussed in Chapter 9. Many riders in equestrian sport overestimate how hard their horses are working, and this easily results in overfeeding.

To evaluate whether your horse is overweight, just right, or underweight you can get him weighed in a clinic the next time you visit. You can also search the internet and find protocols for equine body scores. Do also ask an independent person for their opinion.

> ## Research: glucosamine joint supplements
>
> There is a study from one of the world's leading vet schools, at Guelph in Canada, of (supposedly) glucosamine-based joint supplements. The scientists did lab tests of the contents of some ten different joint supplements to see if the glucosamine level stated was correct. It showed that some producers sold products where what was stated on the container and the actual contents did not match. Some products had a lower glucosamine content than advertised; some had higher, and for one producer the amount of glucosamine in the supplement was zero!

FEEDING, SUPPLEMENTS AND WATER

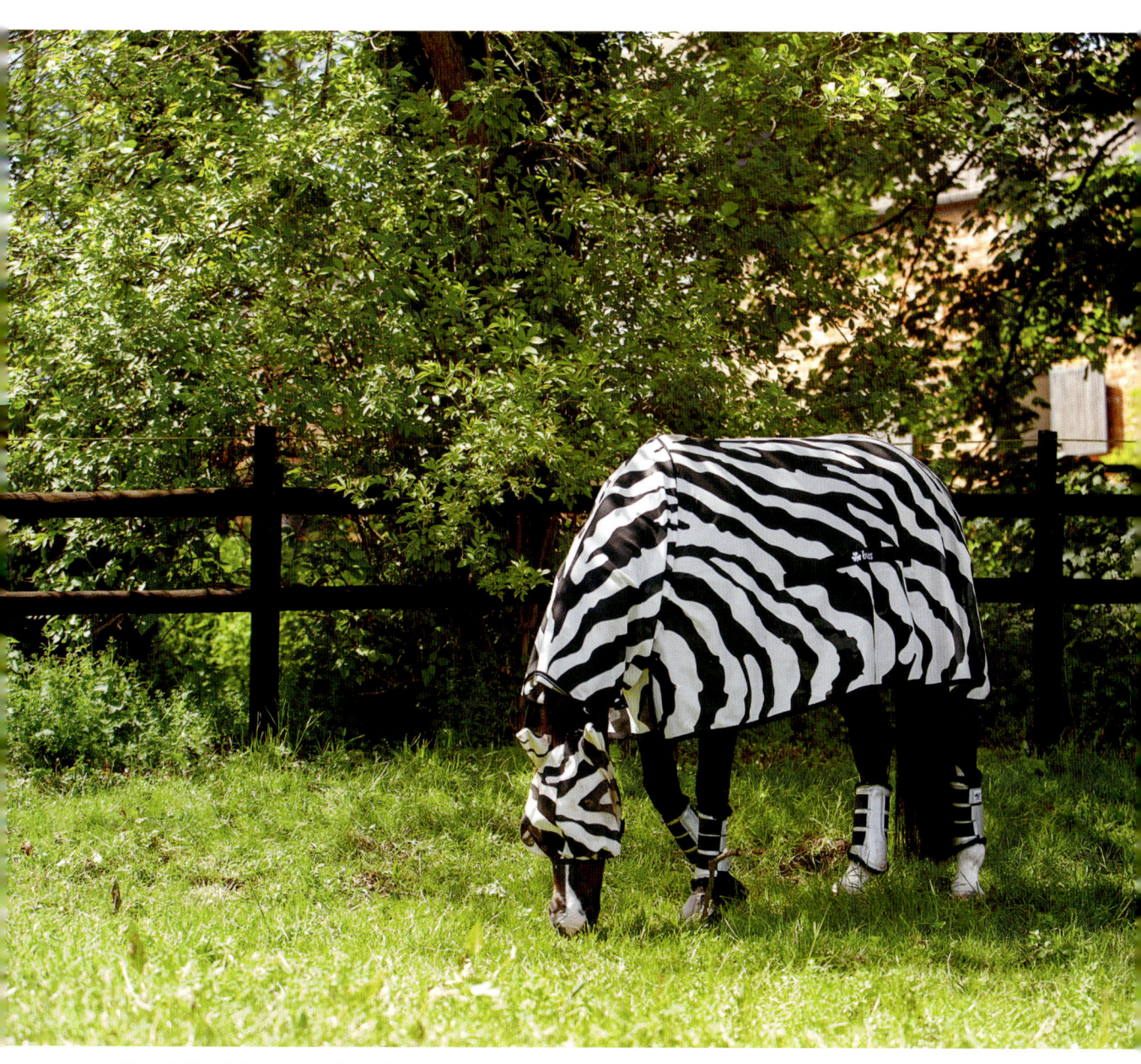

Olympic, World, European and World Cup Champion Valegro on pasture at home. The horses in Carl Hester's yard have daily paddock time. Note, in addition to the insect protection, also the protective boots and the well-built fencing. (*Photo: Jon Stroud.*)

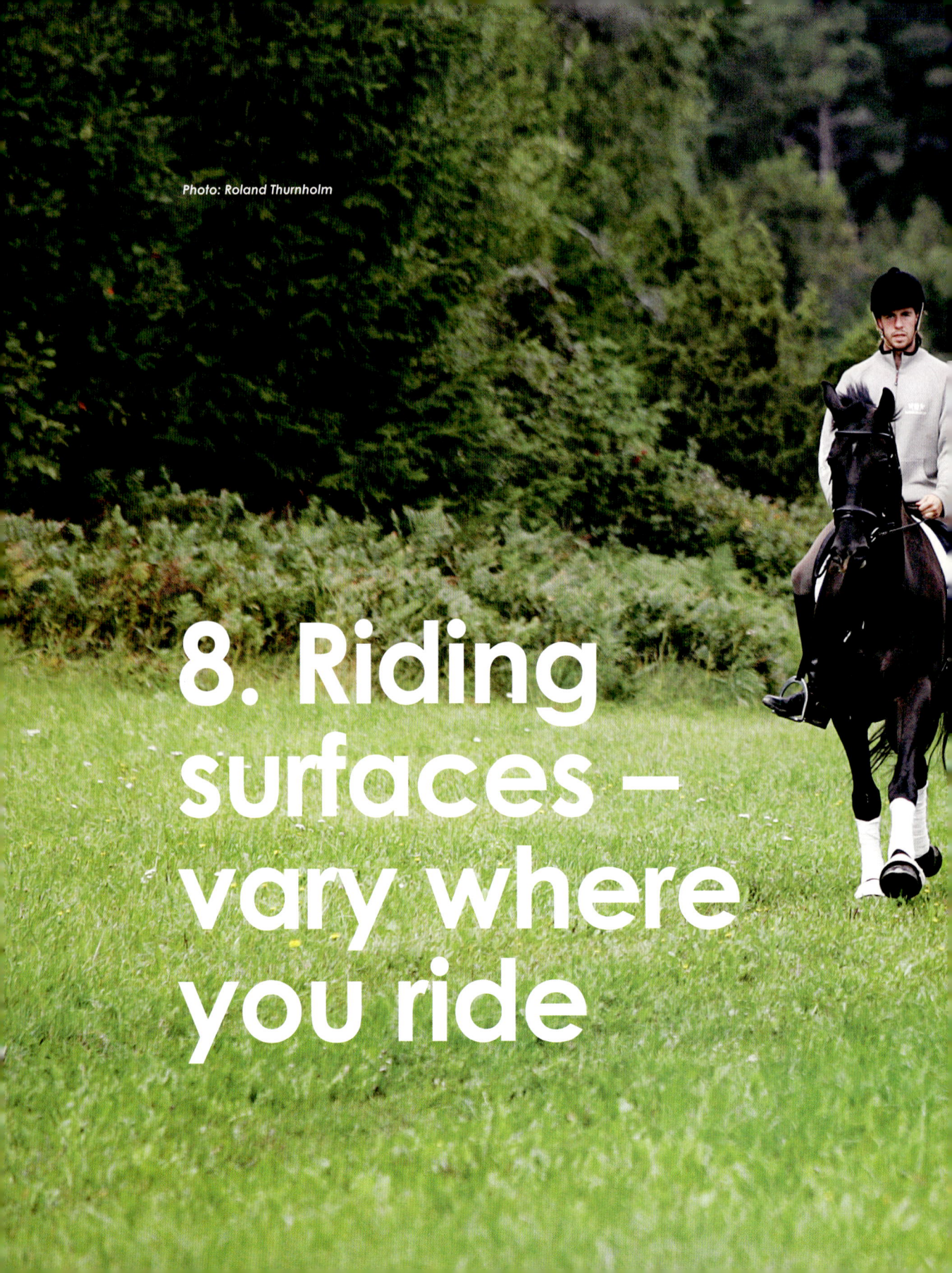

Photo: Roland Thurnholm

8. Riding surfaces – vary where you ride

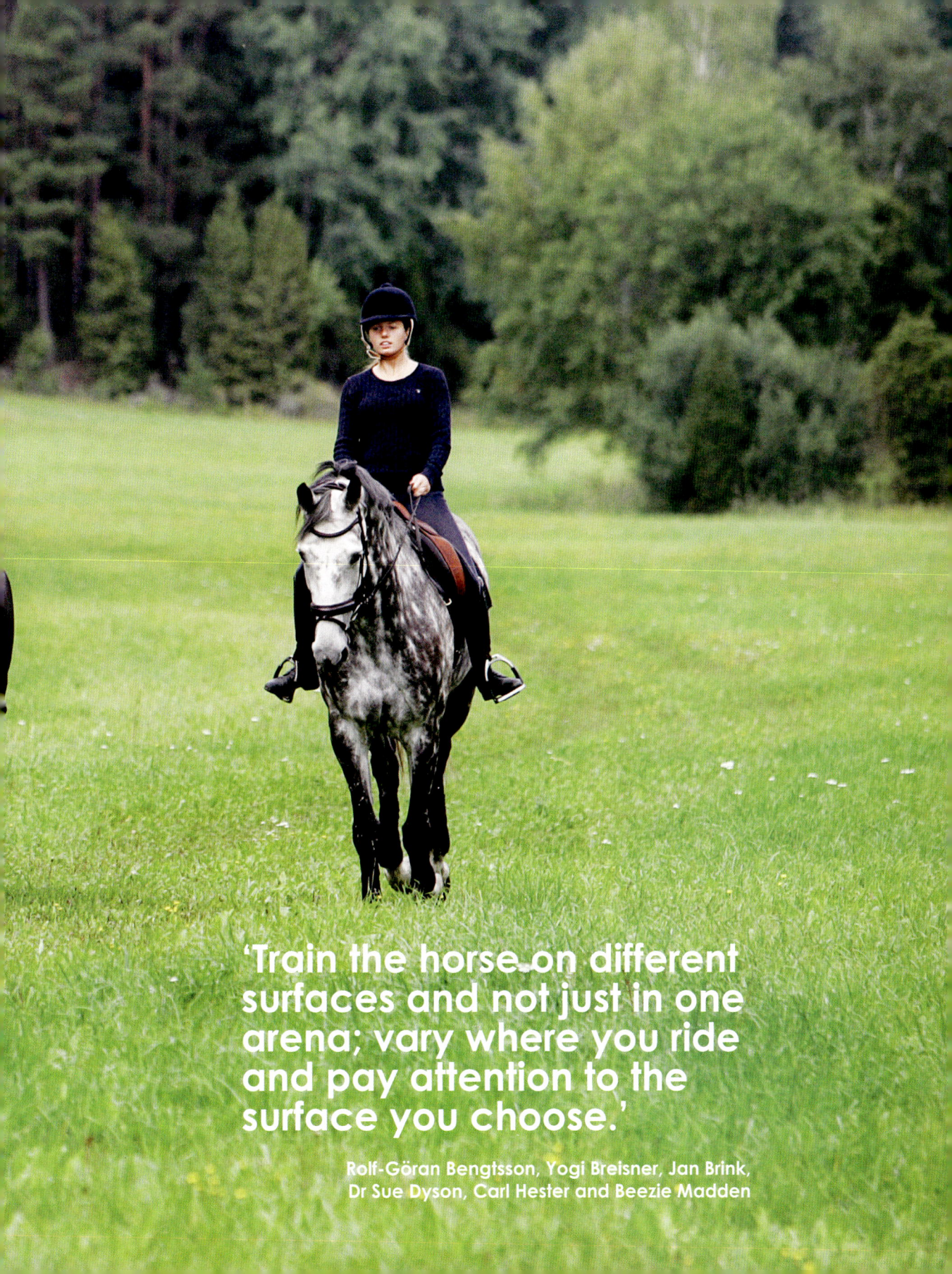

'Train the horse on different surfaces and not just in one arena; vary where you ride and pay attention to the surface you choose.'

Rolf-Göran Bengtsson, Yogi Breisner, Jan Brink, Dr Sue Dyson, Carl Hester and Beezie Madden

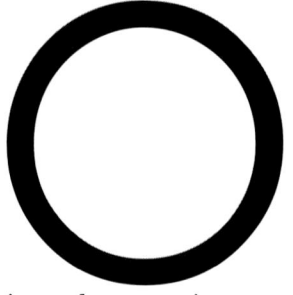

One of the key messages from champion riders and vets concerns the riding surface – pay attention to it and give the horse variety. Both racehorse research and experience has long shown that one important risk factor for injury is the surface the horse trains/competes/races on. This risk is, at the same time, something the rider can influence through knowledge and common sense.

As most people in equestrian sport know, discussions and opinions on surfaces have been very subjective, but research in the past decade has made objective testing possible. It has since been a valuable tool in preparations for the equestrian arenas at the 2012 and 2016 Olympics.

Scientific testing of equestrian surfaces was first developed within Thoroughbred and Standardbred racing, where for decades scientists have studied associations between orthopaedic injury and surface properties.

The FEI and World Horse Welfare helped finance pioneering work on testing and profiling of riding surfaces, at the Swedish University of Agricultural Sciences, undertaken by Professor Lars Roepstorff and his Ph.D student, now Dr Elin Hernlund. They developed an equestrian version of a 'mechanical hoof', called OBST (Orono Biomechanical Surface Tester) originally developed for racecourse testing by Professor Mick Peterson at the University of Maine.

The evaluation points for arenas are:
- Impact firmness.
- Cushioning.
- Grip.
- Responsiveness.
- Uniformity and consistency.

SURFACE CHARACTERISTICS AND USE

Think about how your arena, outdoor and/or indoor, scores on these criteria. At the same time note that a person cannot judge, for example, hardness accurately, because the interaction of the horse and a surface will be different than between a much lighter human and the same surface. Even if you and others feel you have the 'perfect' riding surface, make a point of not riding there all the time. This might sound odd, but it is the same advice as given by the champion riders and by vets. If the horse is ridden constantly on the same surface his body will not be prepared for any variations, and this is suspected to increase the risk of injury.

When jumping riders talk of a 'good surface' at shows they often mean one that allows fast jump-offs; one that is firm and with excellent grip. But firmness and a high degree of grip at the same time increases the load on the horse's legs and could thus increase the injury risk. So what is 'good' for individual performances can be different from what is 'good' for the horse. A non-scientific survey among top names in showjumping in 2014 showed that, at that high level, a majority had elected not to have competition-style surfaces at home. Instead, they had chosen surfaces with less grip and more elasticity than some typical competition surfaces.

To get more surface variation you can consider your surroundings at home and how you can plan your riding so that the horse gets to use different types of surfaces. Do you have access to forest/cross-country riding? Bridlepaths? Grassland?

One important expression in connection with surface use is that 'speed kills'. In this context that means the effect of a surface increases at higher speeds and with jumping. This underlines the importance of using different surfaces in different ways. The higher the speeds you ride at (and also when you are jumping), the more important it is that the surface is even, uniform and has elasticity. But the horse will

> **Reading suggestion**
>
> As with feeding, riding surfaces present a very important subject for the rider to have an understanding of. This chapter is only a short background. The following handbook includes a wide range of information on surfaces. It was published in 2014, first in Swedish, commissioned by the Swedish Equestrian Federation with this author and Dr Elin Hernlund as main co-writers together with an international reference group: http://inside.fei.org/system/files/Equestrian_Surfaces-A_Guide.pdf
>
> For more in-depth background on biomechanics and surfaces, European and US equine surface scientists produced a white paper on surfaces, also published on the FEI website.

also benefit from, for example, riding on uneven terrain, to develop co-ordination and balance – but then at slow speeds.

Just as the body adapts to training, it will also adapt to different surfaces. Compare the effect on yourself if you normally do cross-country running and then suddenly decide to do a session on tarmac. Then, you will probably get sore shins. Among top-level international riders it is now increasingly common to prepare for big classes and especially championships by choosing shows with the same type of surface as at the bigger event.

MAINTENANCE

Irrespective of which arena types you have access to, their maintenance will have great influence on their properties. 'It does not matter what material you put in [on an arena] if it is not maintained properly', Ludger Beerbaum said back in 2007. This is supported by later biomechanical testing of arenas and by footing experts.

Scientific surface testing shows that the same material will offer different properties depending on how it is used and maintained, and that, in turn, different surfaces can share the same properties thanks to appropriate maintenance.

The survey on arena use with top riders in 2014 showed that a majority of them have daily maintenance of their home arenas – and even more than once daily if the arena is in intensive use, as during jumping training.

Opposite: The moisture content of a surface (so how wet or dry it is) is a key factor for its properties. Suitable watering is therefore an important part of maintenance. (Photo: Dr Cecilia Lönnell.)

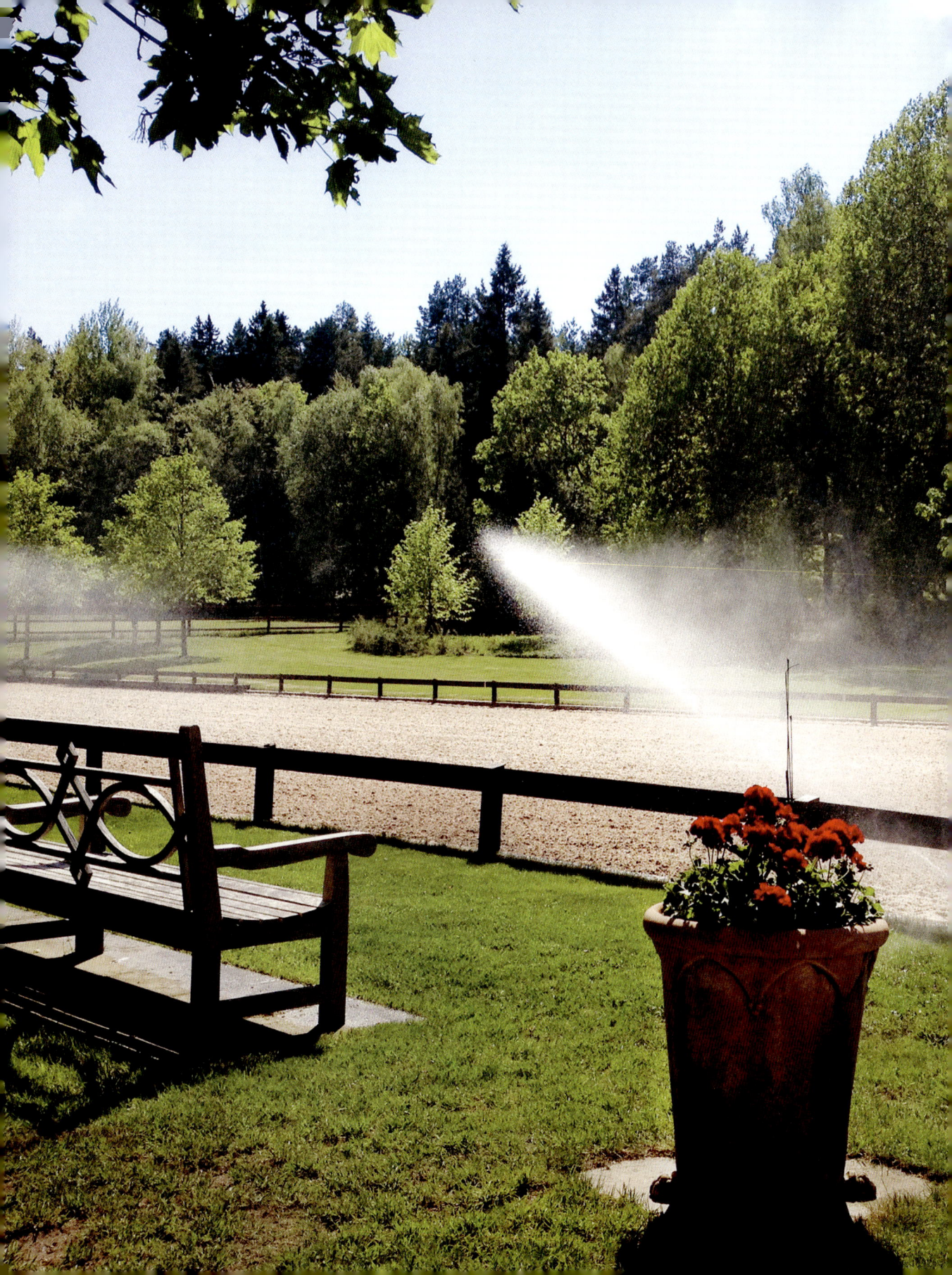

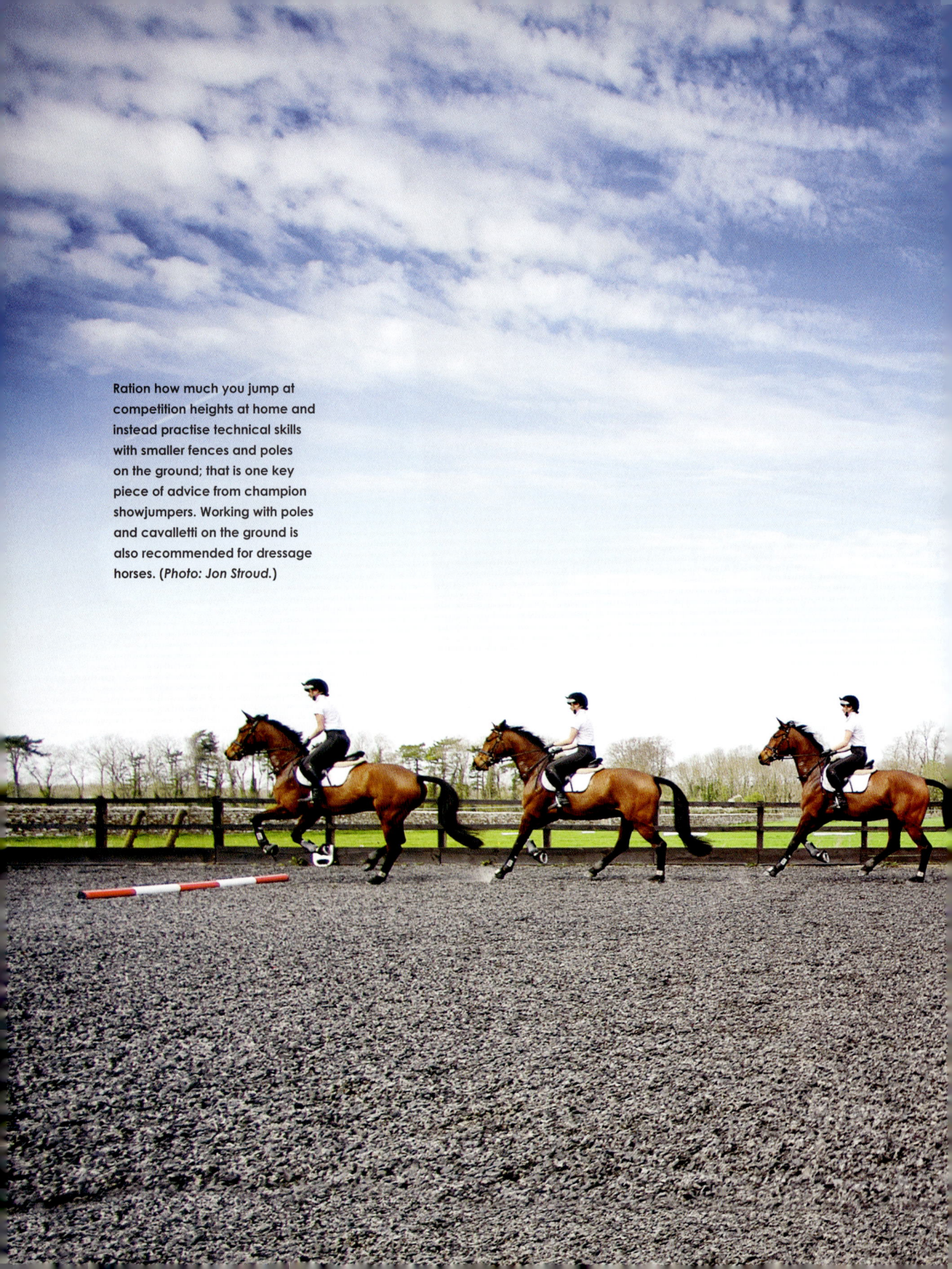

Ration how much you jump at competition heights at home and instead practise technical skills with smaller fences and poles on the ground; that is one key piece of advice from champion showjumpers. Working with poles and cavalletti on the ground is also recommended for dressage horses. (*Photo: Jon Stroud.*)

9. Training

'The guarantee you have when buying a horse lies in the quality of your own training of him, not in how expensive he is.'

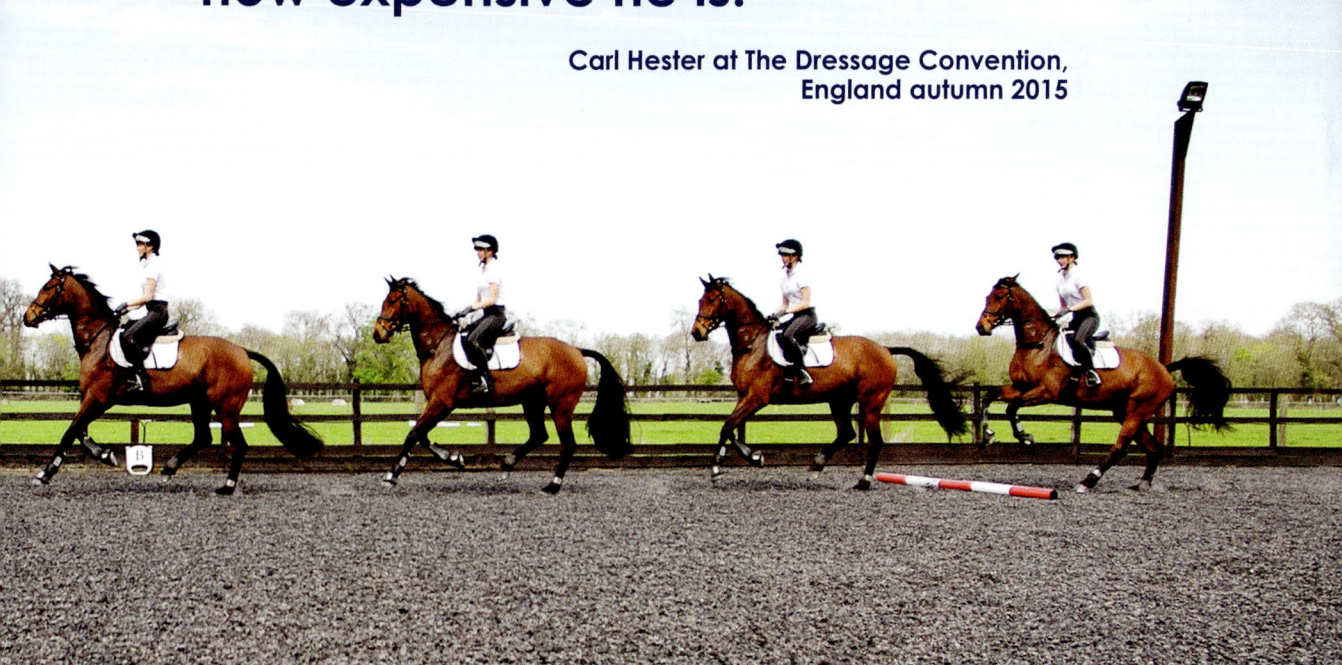

Carl Hester at The Dressage Convention,
England autumn 2015

BASIC TRAINING PRINCIPLES

Champions and other top riders very often stress the philosophy of an ABC of training. This is to start with the basics and get them completely right, and the importance of having a system, a 'thread'. As Ludger Beerbaum and Franke Sloothaak suggest: start by analysing the individual horse and then set up a plan for his training. What can be improved in this horse? Has he been getting too little work, or incorrect work? Is he poorly muscled? Is there something else that needs improving? Such an analysis of course requires experience and skill. Then it is a very good idea to look at the horse together with an experienced coach, and with an experienced horse vet (or speak again to the vet who did the pre-purchase exam if it was recent). Analyse the strong and weak points of the horse, before making any training plans or setting any competition goals. Again, such an analysis can be part of the pre-purchase exam.

Technical training and fitness/conditioning – what is the difference?

Almost all books on riding and training focus on what, in other sports, is called technical training. It is a key factor in all sports: a golfer must practise his putting and his swing; a tennis player his serve and his backhand. It is a question

> 'Give the horse time during training and build him up gradually. Some riders expect that everything has basically already happened. But the horse must be allowed time. You only need to look at yourself if you start a fitness programme. You can't do everything in one go, or else you get sore muscles and aches. And if you then don't allow yourself time to recover it only gets worse.'
>
> Rolf-Göran Bengtsson

of co-ordination, nerve signals and so on. Technical training is, of course, absolutely necessary in equestrian sport – the dressage horse and the rider must master tempi changes, the showjumper must be able to control strides between fences. Technical skills are certainly vital for performance. But many sports today have also realised that, with good physical training, you will improve your technique and performance. When the horse or rider builds fitness through physical training, this also can help prevent injury.

Fatigue is a known risk factor for injury. One reason is that muscles act as a support for joints and tendons/ligaments. When muscles tire this support function diminishes and the load on joints and ligaments and tendons increases. This applies to horses just as it does to the recreational runner.

This is not new knowledge. The body is designed to adapt to higher physical demands, but as we saw in Chapter 2 about the horse's body, that system requires time. Most people know a keen new fitness enthusiast, who ran too far or lifted to heavy weights in his first sessions and quickly got an overuse injury, instead of following a programme where the demands on his body increased more gradually.

How important it is that the horse is allowed to build fitness gradually before being expected to perform was being underlined back at the end of the sixteenth century, at that stage for hunters: 'Of great importance [to avoid injury] is that the hunter is top fit ... this is achieved by a carefully planned training programme where exercise and feeding are increased gradually.' This quote by Gervase Markham is from his (1599) book *How to Chase, Ride, Train and Diet both Hunting Horses and Running Horses*. (Note that this is so early that the Thoroughbred breed did not yet exist).

It is the same philosophy as expressed some ninety years ago by one of Sweden's most legendary equine vets, Professor Gerhard Forsell. In his book *About the horse, its anatomy, care and diseases* (1927) he divided training into 'general' and 'specific':

'The general training has the purpose to improve the fitness of the whole body. The specific training has the purpose to prepare the horse for a specific job. Unfortunately the general training is *often* neglected', he said. (The book was required reading for a rider test developed by the Equestrian Federation.)

The well-known US research vet Dr Hilary Clayton also makes a clear distinction between technical and physical training in her book *Conditioning Sporthorses* (1991). It relates to the same principles as underlined by Professor Forsell. Technical training is basically skills training, including developing a nerve-muscle memory. Conditioning (or what Forsell calls general training) is developing body strength and endurance. Both are necessary in order to have a horse (or athlete) fully prepared for the demands in competition.

It should also be said that the border between technical training and physical training is not always crystal clear. There are dressage exercises that act as technical training but, at the same time, if done correctly, are a form of strength training. Doing transitions is one example; gridwork in jumping is another.

This book is not about technical training, but there is one fundamental technical aspect that we must discuss, as it is so important for long-term results.

Accelerator and brakes

When riders and coaches at the highest level are asked to point out what is the key in all training they underline the importance of first getting the basics, or ABC, right. There are a lot of 'training tips' and exercises around, but most training ideas are a waste of time if the horse and rider have not established correct basics. This is, at the same time, an aspect that many riders below top level are not aware of, or tend to ignore. Go to a clinic with a top rider, and you are almost guaranteed to hear that the 'accelerator and brakes' must function, as the basics for everything else. Below are suggestions from some top names about how to test this at home.

'The better the flatwork is, the better the horse will be over fences', Franke Sloothaak has said. He also underlines that control is important and lack of control is dangerous.

'I realised early on that, in order to succeed in jumping, you need control', John Whitaker said. 'I was lucky when I was young in getting a really good horse in Ryan's Son', John said of his famous partner from the mid-1970s. 'It gave me the chance to compete against the best, and I quickly realised that I did not have the same degree of control as Harvey Smith and David Broome, Hugo Simon or Nelson Pessoa', John said of the time when he was still a Young Rider, 'So I started watching what they did and copied them, a little bit from each. It is really important to have control.'

'So how do you achieve it?', he was asked.

'It is just a question of going back to basics. For example, it is important the horse lands on the correct lead after a fence, that he is straight, and that you can get him back at landing. It is a question of consistent work day after day until the horse understands what you mean. Each time the horse lands he should "come back" to you.'

After Eric Navet of France won double gold medals at the 1990 World Equestrian Games in Stockholm he described his favourite memory as riding John Whitaker's Milton in the four horse change final, as the grey responded so perfectly to the aids, if only two milligrams of extra pressure were applied in each rein. He described it as perfect dressage. When John was later asked how he got Milton so well trained he replied modestly that Milton was like sheepdog who is always asking for his master's next command, but that other horses require more work.

Peter Wylde is one of those who point out that he does not start jumping a horse before the basic flatwork ('accelerator and brakes') is functioning. 'The horse first and foremost needs to learn to respond forwards and to "come back" to you', Wylde said.

Dual Olympic rider Lisen Bratt-Fredricson, wife of Peder Fredricson, spoke in an interview about when Henk Nooren first came to Sweden for a clinic, in which she participated. She and the others were then jumping at 1.30–1.40m level. Lisen had already been training in Holland. Henk set up an exercise to canter between poles on the ground, changing the number of strides within the same distance. This is the same type of exercise that Wylde describes later in this chapter. The riders failed, and Henk declared that he would not return until they could do it. They did their homework, Henk returned, and later became the national team coach, helping Sweden to their best championship results since the 1920s.

Ida-Linn Lundholm and the approved stallion Ampere training at Tullstorp. (*Photo: Krister Lindh.*)

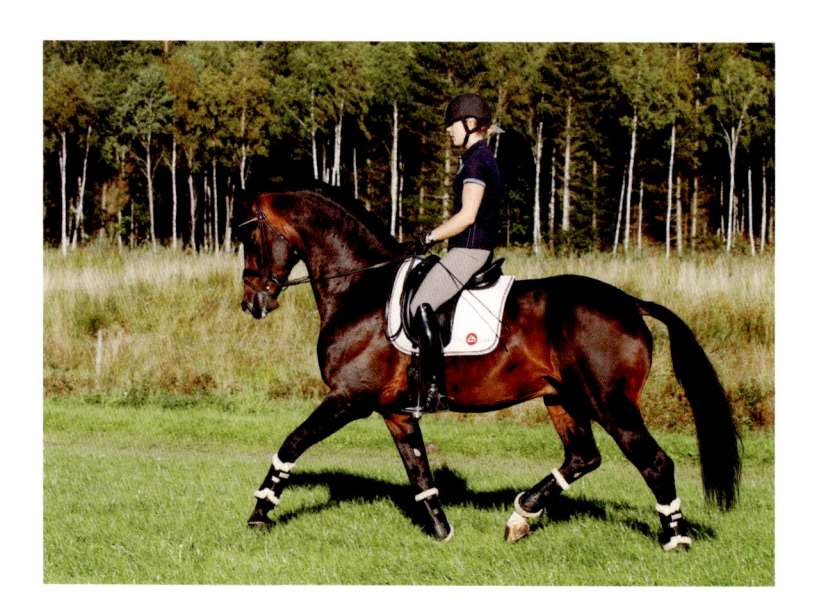

Warming up and cooling down

Apart from going forward and 'braking' there is another kind of basic principle in training that is important to always remember.

It is important that the horse is allowed a warm-up and cooling down period at the start and finish of each training

TRAINING

Test the 'accelerator and brakes' at home!

It is easy for a rider who is riding at home to think that the horse is going great and that 'accelerator and brakes' are working fine. What exercise can you do to test yourself and the horse?

Several riders, including Franke Sloothaak and Beat Mändli, have suggested doing a fast canter on the long side of the arena, and then slowing down and see how that works. 'If you can go faster and slower and the horse stays relaxed that is good!', Franke said. At what level of difficulty you do your exercises should, of course, also be based on how advanced you are right now, he added.

Practising not only distances but also whole course lines just by using poles on the ground instead of fences, or using small fences, is an exercise suggested by Franke and used by many top names. As indicated in Henk's clinic, if you have problems with the lines without fences it will not work any better with fences! 'You should not believe that to jump a 1.40m class you need to practise at 1.60m. That is nonsense!', Franke said.

Peter Wylde gives the following advice:
'What I like to do, and learnt from Henk Nooren, is to set up a line with three not so big fences, say 80–90cm, and vary the distances; 18m plus and just under 22m, and practise riding different numbers of strides. The fences should be low enough so that you can 'play' with the horse.

You can also have two different lines, each with three fences, at 22m and 18m. The 18m distance is of course four strides with bigger fences, but at this height perhaps five or six, and the 22m distance is six strides. What is important is to decide on the number of strides, five, or six, and not ride it and say "Whoa, it was four".

You can do the same on a curved line. Here, too, you must decide beforehand how many strides you will do. It is also important to do it nicely and quietly, without pulling or pushing the horse hard. This exercise helps both horse and rider to understand and learn about speed and rhythm. It is a very useful exercise and you can do it often, let us say every second day. It helps to show whether you and the horse can work together and whether you will be able to ride a whole course or line; ride every stride from the start to the finishing line. Do it on small fences, but with precision.'

Testing the 'accelerator and brakes' is also valid for dressage horses. Kyra Kyrkland and Jan Brink had a dressage clinic at the Stockholm International Horse Show in 2015 where their students had to canter one long side on the arena with different numbers of strides, to practise regulating the canter.

session, Dr Sue Dyson said in her soundness advice. For most fitness enthusiasts and athletes it is a natural part of training to start with a well-planned warm-up period before you begin the real training or competition, and equally to include a cooling down period afterwards. It is regarded as beneficial both for performance and to prevent injury.

Warming up gives the body time to re-route blood flow to the muscles, which then have more oxygen and energy available. Cooling down helps wash away lactic acid, if the horse has done some harder work. The increased body temperature also increases elasticity of muscles, tendons and ligaments.

In equestrian sport you have warm-up arenas at shows, but for some there is less focus on this process at home. But the importance of warming up and cooling down is underlined by names such as Dr Hilary Clayton, Henk Nooren and Carl Hester.

'Carl is very much in favour of the horse getting the chance for a proper warm-up and cooling down. It is good both for the body and mentally', Valegro's groom Alan Davies said in an interview. 'The days when Charlotte works Valegro she rides at 8.00 a.m. So I take him out at 7.30 and hack him for 15–30 minutes, out in the fields or on the lanes around us. Valegro likes saying hello to the neighbour's cows! We have a chat with them across the hedge', Alan said about the now-retired Valegro. After Charlotte's work Valegro then also got a cooling down period.

At the Dressage Convention at Bury Farm in 2015 organised by Carl and Richard Davison, Carl described how when he and Charlotte work their horses it is only 15–20 minutes effective work, with twice that in total for warming up and cooling down.

Carl's and Charlotte's 2012 team gold co-medallist Laura Tomlinson (née Bechtolsheimer) discussed warming up during her demonstration ride at the Dressage Convention:

'When I am warming up I do not ask so much from the horse straight away. I have the whole warm-up to work with; the horse does not need to go perfectly straight away! There are riders who panic if the horse is not going perfectly from the word "go", but it is a mistake, also at competitions, not to let the horse get going a bit, step by step in the warm-up, until you are where you want to be in the arena', Tomlinson said.

Both in showjumping and in dressage top riders say asking too much during the warm-up is a common mistake, especially for showjumpers. Interestingly, UK studies by the Animal Health Trust have shown that while the average warm-up time for elite showjumping riders was 18 minutes the individual strategies varied from 12 to 27 minutes, and (probably unexpected to the riders) doing more work on the left lead than the right. Even at elite level experts have observed that there is a risk of overdoing the warm-up so that the horse 'runs out of petrol' once in the arena. The same group has also studied dressage warm-up and found an average time of some 30 minutes, but shorter at lower levels and longer at higher levels, with indications that warm-up strategies and results were related.

One of Rolf Göran Bengtsson's observations on warming up at shows is that it is important to figure out what type of warm-up fits the individual horse. Some horses need to 'get going'; with other horses it is important to keep them relaxed. It is important that the rider has a set plan for the warm-up and assistance to help realise that.

Training step by step

This book has the title *Sport Horse Soundness and Performance*. We have now come to the core of that theme. In the beginning we looked at seven common causes of injury in athletes: doing too much too soon, lack of continuity, work that is too monotonous, lack of rest and recovery (which includes combining high-volume and high-intensity work), sudden changes in demands or an acute overload incident and individual weaknesses, including re-injury.

A key message in this book is that, from experience, many top riders have a philosophy on training that fits very well with recommendations from human sports scientists to avoid those seven risk situations. That includes a focus on the horse's fitness and physical training and motivation including point one – not doing too much too soon – that the average rider is not aware of.

Franke Sloothaak has underlined that you, as a rider, must have a plan for your work with the horse, an analysis of how he should be brought on and prepared for the demands of competition. Most riders only ride their horse once daily, but it is necessary that the horse gets to be active more than that, and should certainly be outside.

'We must never forget that it is in the horse's nature to be active', Sloothaak said. 'The horse is not born to stand still in a stable. You notice that the more fit a horse gets, the more he wants to do! It is the same with people; the more they get stuck in front of the television, the less energy they get, and the other way around.'

As suggested by Dr Tornell for the Swedish team horses, many top riders have a philosophy of activating the horse in several ways daily. The training plan is not only about a riding session and then standing still inside, or out in a small paddock. Their horses are led and grazed in hand, go in a field or a paddock, are lunged, go on a walker and/or for a light hack.

At first glance this can be difficult to copy for someone with a full-time job outside horses and who is looking after the horse themselves. Also, a high activity level is more of a focus for top horses trained for maximum performances, such as international championships. Still, you can let yourself be inspired to offer the horse more variety in his work, for example by getting assistance from someone who likes to help out with the riding and grooming, leading the horse out for a walk, and choosing a yard that offers facilities such as bigger and better paddocks, a mechanical walker and access to good hacking.

INJURY RISKS AND TRAINING ANTIDOTES*

Common injury risk: Increasing the workload quickly
Antidote: training principle 1 – gradual, stepwise increase in demands

One common injury risk for both horses and fitness enthusiasts/athletes is doing too much too quickly. Rule number one for all training plans is, instead, to increase demands gradually. Franke Sloothaak underlines that a first step in training must be to let the horse build muscles and get physically stronger – what Professor Forsell and Hilary Clayton called general training or conditioning. This requires variation in type, volume and intensity in training – including rest and recovery – listed later on. Step by step the demands then need to increase, otherwise there will be no training effect. When top riders describe how they have developed different top horses they again and again point out that the horse first needed a building-up period, when the body got the chance to build the strength needed for top performance in competition.

Common injury risk: Lack of continuity
Antidote: training principle 2 – be disciplined and make the training planned and regular

Training must be regular and have continuity to have an effect on the body and keep that effect. Occasional sessions at the gym makes little difference in human fitness, but can rather increase injury risk. The same thing holds for horses. Without continuity, fitness and training effect will remain at a low level.

One example of a regular training plan (plus variety, that we will look at in the next point) is from the interview with

*The training principles are frequently cited for human athletes and written for human athletes, but can also be applied to horses, as four-legged athletes. We have used examples from equine research and champion riders' advice mentioned earlier in the book to illustrate this.

SPORT HORSE SOUNDNESS AND PERFORMANCE

Five voices about extended trot – ration it!

Extravagant movement and especially extended trot is appreciated by dressage audiences and judges, but how do they affect the horse? Jan Brink, in his soundness bullet points in Chapter 3, Eric Lette the former head of international dressage judges, and experienced sport horse vets have the same opinion; the inborn talent of modern dressage horses can tempt the rider to ask too much too soon (and too often). Extended trot is one prime example. Professor Gerhard Forsell said the same back in 1927, in his book quoted earlier: 'To work a horse in extended trot before he has come far enough in his training to have the strength to carry the rider in a balanced way at a walk and slower trot, is like driving a heavily loaded wagon at high speed with no suspension. That is, as everyone knows, damaging to the wagon.'

Eric Lette said in an interview that, in his view, extended trot is among the most demanding exercises that are asked of a dressage horse, except for piaffe and passage: 'This is something I have preached but is often forgotten with young horses today, when there is so much focus on spectacular gaits. Riders just push and push.'

Jan Brink's bullet point advice on soundness includes rationing trot extensions. 'If Briar, for example, had done three classes in a weekend and done nine extended trots of 60m each in total he needed to rest and recover both mentally and physically. There are only so many extended trots you can get from a horse', he said.

Professor Lars Roepstorff at the Swedish University of Agricultural Sciences is an expert of equine biomechanics and makes the same point: 'Biologically the principle is always to increase demands gradually. When you do extensions, start with only a few steps and on a good surface. One guideline is to avoid extremes. You should not ask the horse to make too much of an effort for too long, because then the injury risk increases dramatically.'

Professor Forsell discussed extended trot in a chapter of his book concerning injuries and how to prevent them in young horses, writing: 'It is sadly extremely common that the rider does not have enough sense or enough feel not to ask more from the horse than his current level of training allows without overstrain.'

Over eighty years after Forsell's warning, Dr Rachel Murray's research group at The Animal Health Trust in Newmarket had a look at horse's legs in extensions versus collected trot. Their conclusion included the same warning as from Forsell, Brink, Lette and Roepstorff. Her group is interested in possible risk factors for suspensory ligament injury in dressage horses. They started with a small study of four horses and did high-speed filming of horses trotting. Their interpretation was that the suspensory ligaments were subject to higher strains in extensions than in collected trot. 'In the dressage world young horses are expected to show extensions for commercial reasons, but then must also have [had the chance to develop] enough muscle strength not to overload the legs', the group said.

Valegro's groom Alan Davies at Carl Hester's yard. When Valegro was competing he worked in the arena four days a week; Monday, Tuesday, Thursday and Friday. He was hacked and did other outdoor work two days and rested one day.

In the study of elite showjumping riders, which I describe in the next section about training plans, continuity was not analysed. But it was clear from yard visits, interviews and training diaries that these professional riders had a system and a plan for their horses. Even if the systems varied, as we will see later on, almost all had a common thread in what they did during a week, a month or a season. They had a plan for each horse or the yard, instead of being governed by the weather, 'lack of time' or other demands. To achieve that, you need to set up a plan for the horse for the coming week and for the coming months. The exception to when changes should be made in that plan is what several champion riders mention in their bullet point advice in Chapter 3; if the horse seems off-colour.

Common injury risk: Repetitive work
Antidote: training principle 3 – variety

One common cause of injury is repetitive work. Think overuse injuries in the workplace. This can be prevented by variation in training, both in terms of the type of work and the demands made (so intensity and volume). This is also called periodisation. I will come back to that in the next point, about rest and recovery.

Variety is necessary anyway in order to get a complete training plan. Depending on the discipline and the level you compete at, the horse needs different degrees of lung capacity, muscle strength, endurance, co-ordination and nerve-muscle skills, suppleness and mental preparation. This cannot be achieved by only one or two types of activities. Xenophon recommended 2,400 years ago that the rider should vary the riding sessions based on length and location.

Research: training variation reduced injury risk

The international study of showjumping training showed that training variation was the single most influential factor regarding lost training days. The more variety the rider had in the training, the fewer days lost to injury in his horses. In general, riders who did the most flatwork (as a percentage of all training) had the least variety. Hacking out (in the forest/on fields/on lanes) was an important factor in achieving variety. The percentage of hacking out of total training time varied between riders from under five per cent to 47 per cent of the total training. Fitness work was, in general, also part of a varied training programme.

Another indicator that training variation appears to aid soundness is a Ph.D study by Åsa Braam at the Swedish University of Agricultural Sciences, based on analyses of horses who participated in the Quality Testing of four-year-old Warmbloods, and Swedish Federation competition results. Horses who, as youngsters, competed in more than one discipline as a mean had longer careers.

Jos Lansink and his Belgian colleague Ludo Philippaerts both bought land to build their equestrian centres close to a forest and riding tracks, to allow hacking and canter work. John Whitaker, on the other hand, was brought up in hilly Yorkshire countryside ideal for varied riding. 'When my brothers and I grew up we did not have anything except the hilly country around us for riding. We only had a small outdoor arena and it was on a slope, so we mainly hacked out and used the hills, and realised that it worked', he said.

The Swiss Olympic and World Cup Champion Steve Guerdat said in an interview that he found a way to vary his training. In the same way as some people load their horses on a lorry to get to an indoor arena he, on a weekly basis, took a few of his horses to an area with excellent riding terrain.

Carl Hester's bullet point advice in Chapter 3 also includes not always riding in an arena: 'Don't practise dressage exercises the whole time, because that will mean wear and tear on the horse. That they do not only do dressage work is also good for their mentality. Fitness work is important. We have hills at home where we work them to develop muscles and cardiovascular fitness.'

Beezie Madden's advice on training variation is very similar to Carl's, John's and other colleagues: Hack out in varied terrain, let the horse go in the field (grass), do flatwork and have them on a walker.

Common injury risk: Lack of rest and recovery – combining intensity and volume
Antidote: training principle 4 – periodisation

Lack of recovery time is also on the list of common injury risks. One antidote is what in sports science is called periodisation. It means varying between harder and lighter work and including breaks for rest and recovery. Lack of recovery and too much hard training will, in the end, lead to overtraining or what, in the human workplace, is called burnout.

TRAINING

Dr Clayton advised on including rest days in a training plan and against doing strenuous work two days in a row. This fits with racehorse study results indicating, for example, that the suspensory ligament tendon is subject to microdamage after intense exercise, which is reversible (so will repair itself) after a few days. Reflect on what would happen if the horse and his tendon are subjected to further intense work before the repair process is finished.

Remember:
It is very important to differentiate between:
1. planned rest days, as part of a training plan

in contrast to:
2. The horse losing a training day when he was meant to be in work because you were tired or short of time.

'Rest' is not just standing still in a stable or small paddock, but also being led out in hand, or light hacking.

Research: The importance of recovery

One example of the importance of recovery in supporting soundness is found in a study of orthopaedic injury in Swedish riding school horses. Horses in a group of riding schools with very low numbers of orthopaedic injuries as a mean had longer summer grazing periods (on pasture 24/7 with no riding).

Research: does the horse exercise himself in a paddock?

Some European countries, including Sweden, have laws on horses having to be allowed out in the field or a paddock. But is this equivalent to any exercise? An Australian research group including B.M. Hampton, whose main study subject was wild horses, tested GPS-senders on a group of domestic horses to study how much they move around. They found an association between the size of the paddock or field and the horse's level of activity in a day. In a 20 x 40m paddock the horse moved very little. In a field of 16 hectares (an area equivalent of 32 soccer pitches) the study horses moved a mean of 7.5km per day. If your only option is a small paddock where the horse will be quite passive, remember that this study indicates that even if the horse has been out all day he has not had any real exercise. Also remember that he might want other, mental stimulation. Leading the horse out in hand is one idea. Walkers are not liked by all horses, but offer slow exercise as a complement.

SPORT HORSE SOUNDNESS AND PERFORMANCE

Check the horse's legs daily!

One advice about minimising injury problems is to give the horse your own daily check-up, especially palpating the legs. The aim is to spot and address any problems early. Is there any swelling or heat? Any soreness? You can ask your vet or an experienced professional to teach you.

Opposite: John Whitaker is one of those champion riders who believes in giving the horses a varied training regimen. Here he is on Milton at his farm in Yorkshire. (*Photo: Bob Langrish.*)

How does the body respond to training? Adaptation signalling

There are two very important principles for the body's adaptation to training, which you should have in mind when planning either a single training session or a whole plan, involving specific training.

One is that, to get a training effect, the effort must reach a certain threshold or level, otherwise the body will not register a signal for adaptation. Imagine that you lift or carry a small bag of potatoes, compared to a sack of potatoes. The small bag will give no training effect as the body is used to the lighter weight. This threshold will change as the body's fitness changes.

The other principle for training and adaptation is that, once the body has registered a strong enough signal, it will respond and start the adaptation process, but then shut it down again quite quickly, even though the exertion continues. This underlines the important difference between quality and quantity in training. One example is a study on bone adaptation, where rats were made to jump as an exercise to improve bone strength. The finding was that five jumps had the same effect on bone formation as twenty jumps. Of course the five jumps meant less wear and tear than twenty.

Consider this in relation to horses and training; a showjumper needs to jump fences of a certain height as a preparation for competition, but after a few jumps the body will shut off the adaptation signal. From then on more jumps at that height will only give more wear (to allow for more technical training, use poles on the ground or small fences).

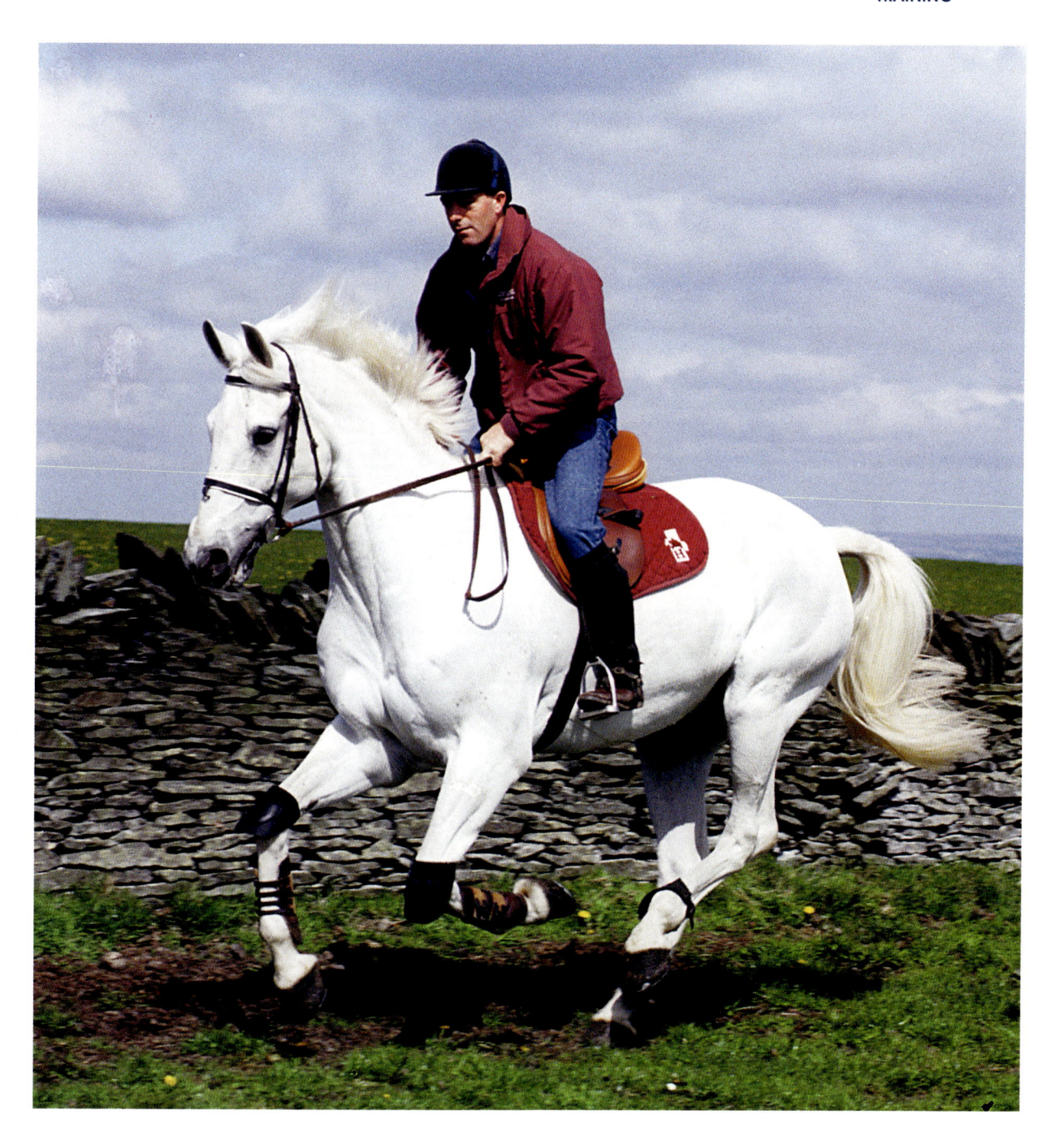

TRAINING

SPORT HORSE SOUNDNESS AND PERFORMANCE

The horse is born to eat grass!

Several champion riders in this book underline the importance of the performance horse being happy and content, and being allowed to express natural horse behaviour as part of sound management.

In 2010, at the ISES conference at Uppsala, famous sport horse vet Sue Dyson recommended as part of injury prevention that the horse should get recovery time through regular free exercise and 'playtime'; time in the field and on a walker are probably beneficial, she said.

In Sweden a horse, by law, must be allowed out several hours a day and be able to move at walk, trot and canter, but the rules do not mention the type of ground in the field or paddock. Sweden has a law about mandatory summer grazing for cows. Both are grazing animals, but for some unexplained reason there are no legal rules saying a horse must also be allowed to graze.

Many countries do not have any such regulations. In a query with FEI Top Ten riders, nine had their horses out in a field or paddock at home, and eight out of ten had them on grass (with some individual horses as exceptions). Those not let out on grass were grazed in hand.

The horses out in grass paddocks included stars bought or valued at five to ten million euros or dollars, such as Jeroen Dubbeldam's European and World Champion Zenith SFN.

One main argument from, for example, Steve Guerdat and Beezie Madden for this choice is that horses are grazers by nature and have an inborn need to express that instinct. With some of the world's best horses the rider and/or groom describes grazing in the field as the horse's favourite pastime.

Peder Fredricson offered the following analysis: 'In my opinion, if a horse, already warmed up from riding, is then put in a correctly designed paddock but cannot handle that, then he probably cannot handle jumping a course either', he said.

When these top horses are let out it is with the same attention to detail as in training; well-built fencing, well-maintained grounds without stones, and with protective boots on.

Elsewhere in the book we will look at dressage horses and time in the field. The now-retired Olympic, World and European Champion Valegro was allowed that (as are the other horses in Carl Hester's yard), and the same was true of Jan Brink's multiple medallist stallion Briar, and more and more top dressage riders seem to follow that example.

TRAINING

The horses in the showjumping study had, in general, at least one planned rest day per week. Some riders also gave their younger horses (under seven years) a summer grazing period after the season's most important young horse championships. (Summer grazing means being in the field without work.)

Beezie Madden has described giving her horses about two months winter break, when they go in the field without shoes 'being horses'. Rodrigo Pessoa used to time the now-legendary Baloubet du Rouet's annual break in late spring, in a grass paddock (with high fencing). Pessoa has said that important parts of the management of Baloubet concerned keeping him relaxed and in a good mood. (Rolf Göran Bengtsson's bullet point advice in Chapter 3 also includes the importance of the horse being relaxed).

One example of individual differences in the same yard was supplied by dressage legend Anky van Grunsven at the EEHNC in 2015. Her Olympic Champion Salinero only went into a field twice in his whole career, and one of those times he injured himself so that he missed the European Championships, because he was so explosive. He was, however, taken out to graze in hand every day. His stablemate Bonfire, in contrast, went in a grass paddock some three hours a day.

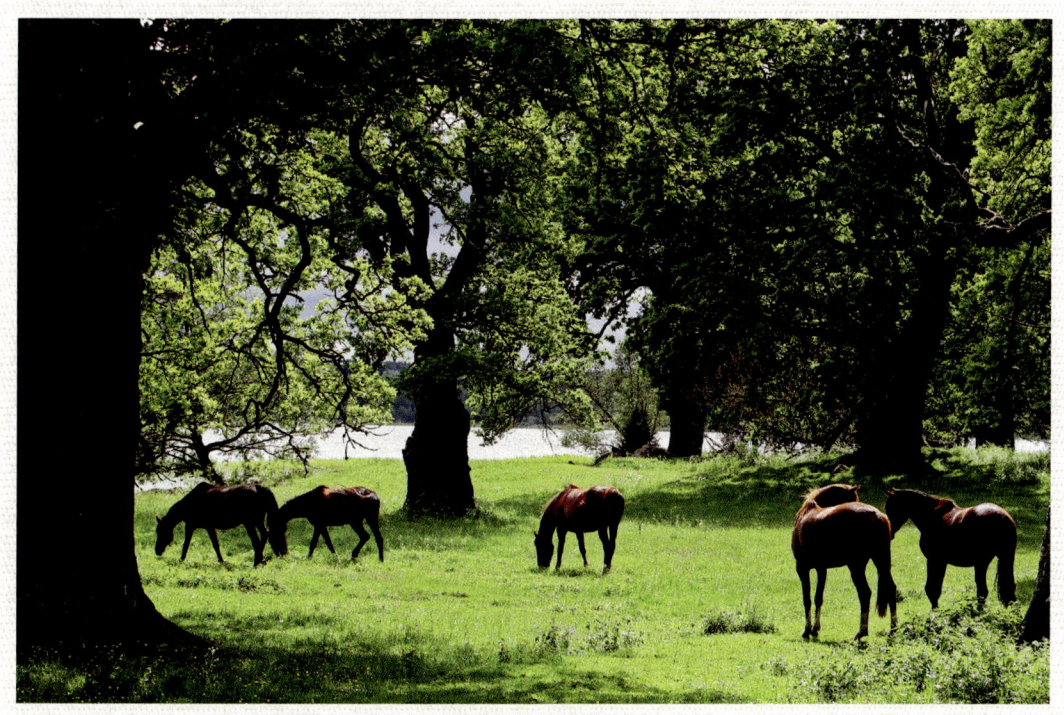

School horses on pasture at the National Equestrian Centre at Strömsholm. (*Photo: Roland Thunholm.*)

To focus further on the principle of periodisation, it means that you must vary the demands in training over the year, and ration your competitions – this is what Rolf Göran Bengtsson, Yogi Breisner, Jan Brink and Dr Jonas Tornell refer to when talking about the importance of planning the season.

One important example is not to combine lots and hard work at the same time (so balance intensity and volume of work). This is important to remember when planning fitness work; it should be planned in preparation for important competition periods and not *during* them. Both Jonas Tornell and Franke Sloothaak suggest winter as a time to start building fitness:

'In the summer there will be competitions. Then you do not have time to develop the horse physically, instead use winter for that, and also to get the horse stronger and more supple through gymnastics. The better prepared the horse is before the season starts in earnest, the better he can perform', Franke said.

Interval training

One example of periodisation is interval training, well known from human sports training but also for racehorses. It can be applied in most types of intensive training. For example, instead of doing a 1,000m canter you let the horse do 2 x 500m, with a short rest in between. Gridwork jumping can also be a type of interval training, for example jumping one grid, a rest and then jumping the grid again, or doing eight jumps in one go and then eight again, rather than sixteen without interruption. Interval training has the advantage that the athlete or horse does intensive work, but with recovery periods, which prevents the fatigue that easily accumulates in a non-stop session.

Even though it would not count as interval training as such, you can also use the idea in a flatwork or dressage session by giving the horse plenty of mini-breaks at walk. This is one of Jan Brink's bullet points (see Chapter 3) – do not tire the horse by long uninterrupted trotting or cantering work.

Common injury risk: Sudden change in demands, or sudden overload
Antidote: training principle 5 – specific training = practise competition demands

A sudden change in demands on the body is a common injury risk, closely related to the dangers of a fast increase in training. This point includes sudden overload, such as may result in an accidental sprain.

One example of a sudden change in demands is if the horse has not performed in training what he is expected to do in competition. While a training programme should be varied, it must also include the specific demands in competition (after first having the building-up period we discuss in training principle 1). As we will see in the examples of the racehorse study later in this chapter, specific training does *not*, however, mean that the showjumping horse should jump courses at competition height day after day, as Beezie Madden points out, or that a Grand Prix dressage horse should be doing piaffe and passage day after day at home. The UK racehorses who do so-called fast work at home (to practise race speeds) do it at shorter distances than in the actual race and a maximum of twice a week!

Common injury risk: Individual weaknesses, including previous injuries
Antidote: training principle 6 – pay attention to the horse's individual response

In all training it is important to remember that every horse will respond differently to the same training regimen. As Rolf Göran Bengtsson, Ludger Beerbaum, Franke Sloothaak and others pointed out earlier, this means that it is important to observe how the horse responds to the training, what signals he gives, and adapt your plan to that. Having that feel is what in farming is called an 'animal eye'.

As I said earlier, there are many factors that influence

the training response, such as genes (breeding), previous training, temperament and motivation. Do remember that previous injuries are an important risk factor for new injuries! This is the background of Dr Tornell's bullet point advice in Chapter 3 – to try to avoid injuries and setbacks in young horses, in order to improve their chances of a long career. Every horse benefits from having his own plan: not all individuals can be worked in the same way.

Some ninety years ago Professor Gerhard Forsell said it was important to pay attention to the horse's signals in training, and respond if the horse, for example, showed resistance.

In the international showjumping study a majority of the participating elite riders had a low percentage of days lost to training because of injury or disease – some, basically none. Yard vets of the Swedish riders confirmed this pattern – i.e. that they had fewer problems than the average, maybe amateur rider. Their impression was that the elite riders were better than average at feeling and responding to changes in the horse. A small injury could then be addressed simply by some rest. A very similar reflection about the importance of observing and responding to the horse's signals – for example, lack of enthusiasm or resistance – was pointed out by experienced riding school professionals in the riding school horse study.

TRAINING PLANNING

We have looked at how the body's bone, joint cartilage, tendons and ligaments respond to training and what training regimens can lessen or increase the risk of injury. Champion riders have given some advice based on their experience. As Franke Sloothaak said in the beginning of the book, it is very important to have a plan for the horse and follow it.

In order to make a training plan the rider first needs to analyse what stage or level of training the horse is at right now. The second step is to decide what level you are aiming for and what the physical demands are there. The plan might need to include smaller incremental goals. As we have seen in previous chapters, it is very important that the horse is allowed to develop and build capacity for the job he will he required to do in competition. It is then also important to push 'rewind' if the goal, for some reason, needs adjusting and takes longer than expected to reach. Based on your analysis of the horse's strengths and weaknesses, and depending on what discipline and what level you ride at, the horse needs to develop the following attributes:

Co-ordination – balance and nerve-muscle memory
'Co-ordination is important for the technical performance, but remember also that a horse with poor balance is also more prone to stumbling, and then can also be more at risk of injury', said Dr Clayton.

Suppleness training
Exercises for suppleness have the aim of improving mobility by stretching muscles, tendons and ligaments and flexing joints that determine movement. This is one important reason why it is important to allow the horse warm-up time in the beginning of each training session.

Fitness and muscle strength
Give improved power and endurance.

Training diary
In the European jump training study described in Chapters 1 and 3, the study riders filled in daily training protocols, thus a training diary. Many riders have a notebook in the stable, but it can be quicker and give a better overview to use a standardised form. To set up a training schedule you need to consider four points for every session:

1. What activity?

SPORT HORSE SOUNDNESS AND PERFORMANCE

2. How often?

3. How long?

Nos. 2 and 3 determines the training volume. The third factor is:

3. At what intensity?

You can organise your own training diary on those lines. Equestrian sport is also getting training apps of the same type as for fitness enthusiasts, that simplifies keeping track of and analysing your training.

At what intensity does the sport horse work?

If your aim is to jump a 1.40m class or do a Medium dressage competition, or novice event, do you know what heart rate a fit horse while competing at that level is? Do you know how to check your own horse's heart rate? Have you thought about how you determine the intensity in a training session?

Jumping and dressage riders are, in general, less familiar with judging intensity compared to an event rider or, more so, racehorse trainer. In the European jumping training study the elite riders differed greatly in their evaluation of how close to his maximum possible effort the horse was in a jumping session, or in canter work. Different riders had, for example, very different views on the intensity of a 400m per minute canter session, even with horses of the same age and training level. A German thesis on dressage training came the same conclusion.

A showjumper or dressage horse does not, of course, have to make the same physical effort as a racehorse, or an event horse going cross-country. However, he still needs to build fitness and strength to perform as well as possible at his level and have some reserve capacity. You should remember that the actual competition can include short sequences of higher exertion.

Heart rate monitors

Measuring heart rate is one method of measuring how hard

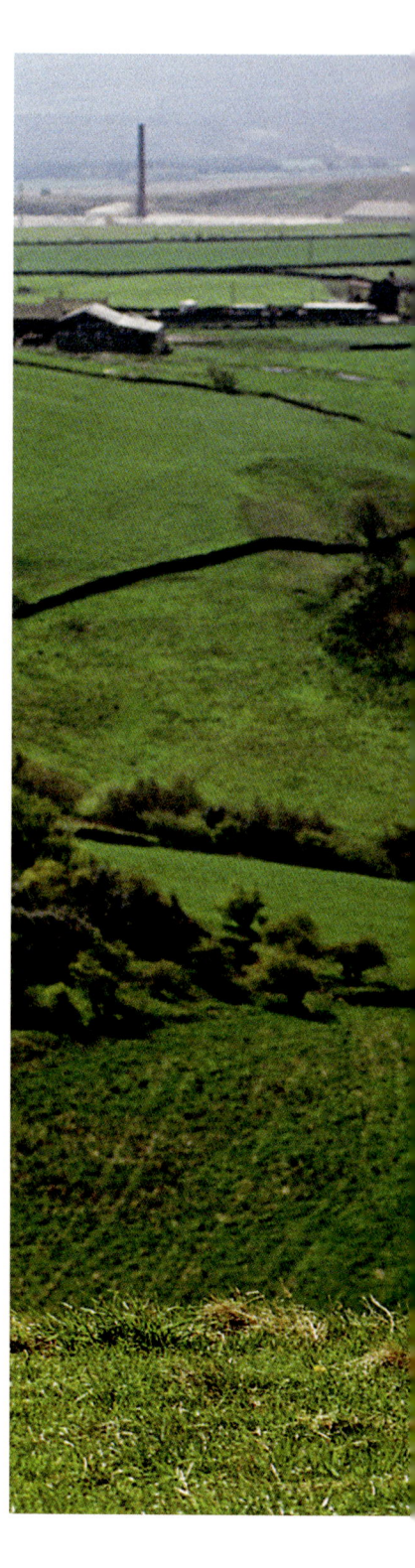

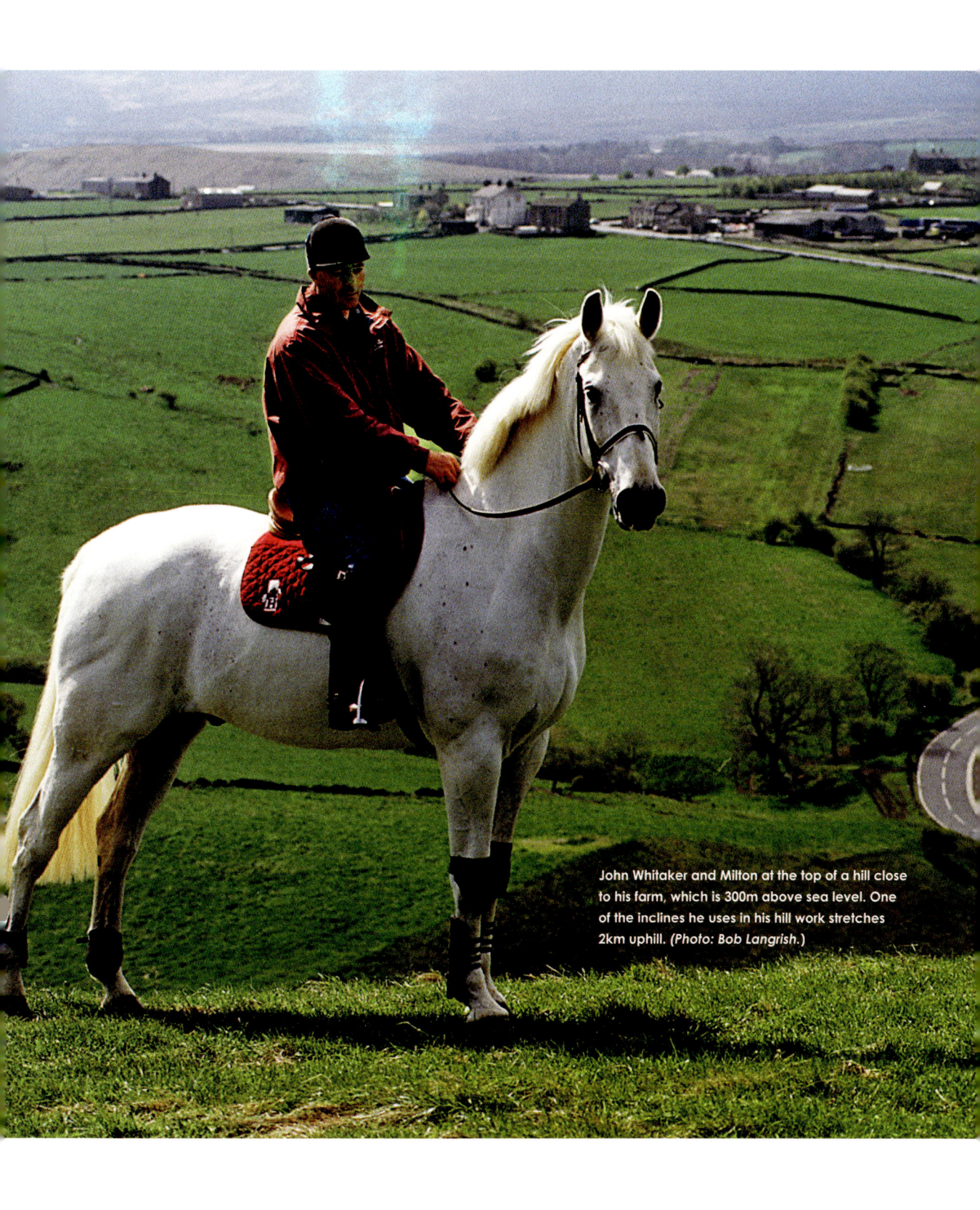

John Whitaker and Milton at the top of a hill close to his farm, which is 300m above sea level. One of the inclines he uses in his hill work stretches 2km uphill. *(Photo: Bob Langrish.)*

a horse is working. It is used more in racing, eventing and endurance than in dressage or showjumping. In endurance, of course heart rate is one factor that determines whether or not the horse is allowed to continue.

A traditional equine heart rate monitor is put around the ribcage, as for a human athlete. The handling requires some getting used to, and patience, but allows a more objective monitoring of fitness training.

To be able to judge the intensity of work better you should be aware of the horse's working heart rate. This is displayed by the heart rate monitor. You will be able to see differences at different speeds, on different surfaces, and with the same work but in different horses – and over time as fitness increases. When you know the normal heart rate at rest of an individual horse, changes will help you detect early signs of infection, as well as pain. Dr Charlie Lindberg and his co-author Ingrid Andersson have suggested the following strategy. (First you must practise feeling the pulse!). Dismount straight after the work you want to measure. The working heart rate will drop quickly, but if you have practised and are quick to detect it, it has probably only dropped by about 25 per cent, they said.

Approximate heart rates by speed/activity

GAIT/ACTIVITY	SPEED	HEART RATE
REST		28–40
SLOW TROT	250 M/MIN	80–130
NORMAL TROT	300 M/MIN	100–150
CANTER	350 M/MIN	120–160
GALLOP	500 M/MIN	150–200
DRESSAGE NOVICE-M		MAXIMUM APPROX 130
JUMPING 1 M		MAXIMUM APPROX 155
JUMPING HIGHER CLASSES		MAXIMUM APPROX 190
CROSS-COUNTRY		170–200
MAXIMUM EFFORT		240

So if you feel 120 beats per minute, the horse will have been working at 150 beats per minute (that is multiply the number of beats by 1.33).

A horse's maximum heart rate is about 240 beats per minute. To even reach 50 per cent of his maximum heart rate a horse needs to canter at 350m per minute or more, and few jumpers or dressage horses do that in training. This, of course, also means that horses have a much higher capacity for work than many riders realise. But – as is pointed out repeatedly in this book – if they are going to be asked to perform more strenuous work they must be prepared for it by appropriate training.

How to you develop your horse's fitness?

The importance of a gradual increase of work in a training process is a key message in this book. It is often overlooked in riding handbooks. The process of bringing an unfit horse to full fitness can be described in three steps, like a staircase.

Step 1: Requires the most time, to build a basic fitness through low-intensity work.

Step 2: Strength training, when the horse develops muscles and more endurance.

Step 3: Fitness work, when the basics are in place.

One example of the positive effect of developing an extra gear comes from a dressage team preparing for a championship in a hot climate. The riders were advised to add 350m/minute canter work to their training. No dressage horse does 350m/minute canters in competition, but several well-known dressage riders both now and in the past have (had) canter tracks at home, or transport(ed) their horses to a racetrack for faster canter work, their feeling being that dressage horses also benefit from canter fitness work. The team horses who did the canter fitness programme reportedly lost some weight, and seemed happier and had more 'petrol' all through three classes, as demanded in a championship.

Before the 2004 Athens Olympics, fitness training was a very important part of the preparation of the Swedish jumping team, that won a team silver medal.

Step 1 – slow outdoor work

Again, the first step is to build basic fitness.

Fundamentally, this starts with hacking out, straight ahead on (quiet) roads or similar, with an even surface. The UK tradition is called roadwork, getting a gradual increase in basic fitness through walk and trot. From day one up to high-intensity work the process takes about three months. Dr Hilary Clayton calls this slow work.

Riding on a road can be the only outdoor choice in many places. But a (quiet) tarmac road also has the advantage of offering a firm, even surface. Dr Hilary Clayton grew up in the UK and feels the ideal surface for this type of training is where the hoof gives some mark, so more a softish gravel road.

Roadwork is sometimes said to have the purpose of strengthening the horse's tendons through the impact of riding on tarmac. But horses in the British Isles did roadwork long before tarmac was laid out.

The idea that roadwork strengthens the superficial digital tendon might be linked to the fact that fatigue and lack of fitness are known risk factors for tendon injury. So a horse who has undergone a roadwork programme before more strenuous work will be fitter and better prepared for more intense work, which increases tendon load! So it is thus the improved fitness that is the protective factor, rather than any beneficial effect on the tendon itself.

Eventing guru Yogi Breisner has made the same observation as scientists studying equine tendons; that a lot of time spent on tarmac causes wear and tear, with police horses as one example. At the same time, he feels that tendons and ligaments can benefit from work on a firm, even surface. Tendons and ligaments are then stretched in a controlled manner.

TRAINING

Below is an example of a roadwork schedule in two well-known National Hunt racing yards. Week one in the table is at the end of the summer. Then, four-year-old horses come in to start their training, and older horses come back from about two months summer break without work. The point here is to show the week by week schedule of a building-up period for horses who have just entered training, or who are coming back from a long rest. How many jumping or dressage riders give their horses six-eight weeks hacking in walk and trot before starting to demand more after a lay-off?

Example of a road work programme

WEEK	TRAINER 1	TRAINER 2
1	walk (6 days)	walk (6 days)
2	walk (6 days)	walk (6 days)
3	walk (6 days)	walk and trot 1 hour
4	walk and trot 1-1.5 hours (6 days)	walk and trot 1 hour
5	walk and trot 1-1.5 hours (6 days)	walk and trot 1 hour
6	walk and trot 1-1.5 hours (6 days)	walk and trot 1 hour
7	trot 6 days (Some horse 3 days x 600m slow canter)	3 days 800m canter 3 days 2,100m canter
8	3 days 600 m slow canter, 3 days trot	6 days canter
9	4 days slow canter, 2 days higher speed	6 days canter
10	6 days canter	6 days canter
11	finish session at racing speed	6 days canter

(Regarding tarmac or not, trainer 1 especially did not use roads but primarily his own excellent grassland)

One British example of a roadwork programme for equestrian use suggests a minimum of at least two weeks at only walk, at first 30–45 minutes, gradually increased to an hour and a half. Racehorse trainer 1's schedule was three weeks of walking only. Another suggestion is to include some inclines after the first few weeks, and introduce trotting little by little, so short distances only at first.

SPORT HORSE SOUNDNESS AND PERFORMANCE

Dr Hilary Clayton recommends six to 12 months building-up period in her book *Conditioning Sport Horses*, but later modified that to about three months, which corresponds to the racing yard examples here.

Swedish vets Dr Charlie Lindberg and Dr Staffan Lidbeck (Sweden's former eventing chef d'equipe and vet) have suggested that six to eight weeks is sufficient to build basic fitness for a horse used for light recreational riding and Novice dressage. Within three months, as in Dr Clayton's plan, you reach the level of faster canter work.

Step 2 – muscle strength/power

'Horses can't, of course, do weightlifting, but irrespective of discipline they need to develop their muscle strength. Hillwork and gridwork seems to have the right effect', said Dr Clayton.

Both she and colleague Dr Rachel Murray at the Animal Health Trust in Newmarket are dressage riders, and both recommend what, in human gyms, is called cross-training, but for dressage horses. One definition of cross-training is that an athlete trains in other activities than their specific sport, with the aim of improving total performance – 'Do not do the same thing every day in training', Dr Clayton advises.

Both she and Rachel Murray also recommend developing strength in the horse's trunk, what in human gyms is called the body core. The more extravagant the horse is in his way of moving, the more core body muscle strength he needs. Well-developed back muscles are one important factor, Dr Clayton said.

For developing core strength, she and Dr Murray recommend working on transitions, using poles on the ground, feeding the horse on the ground (to make him stretch his neck) and riding certain sessions in a long and deep position (not short and deep, or with the head towards the breast as in rollkur). The fact that transitions are a good gymnastic exercise for horses is also pointed out by Carl Hester.

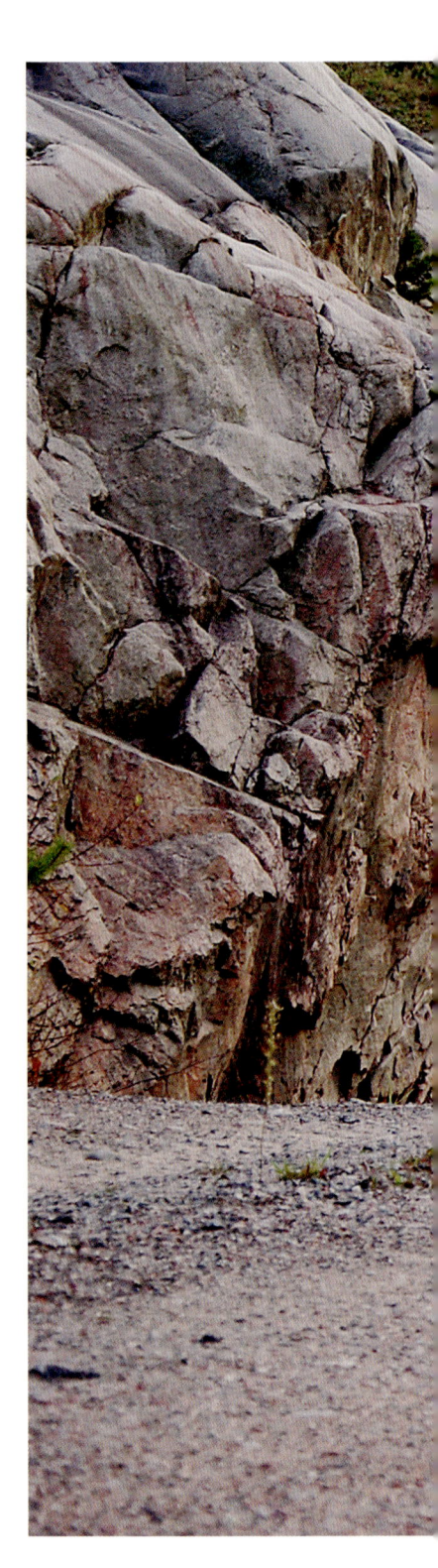

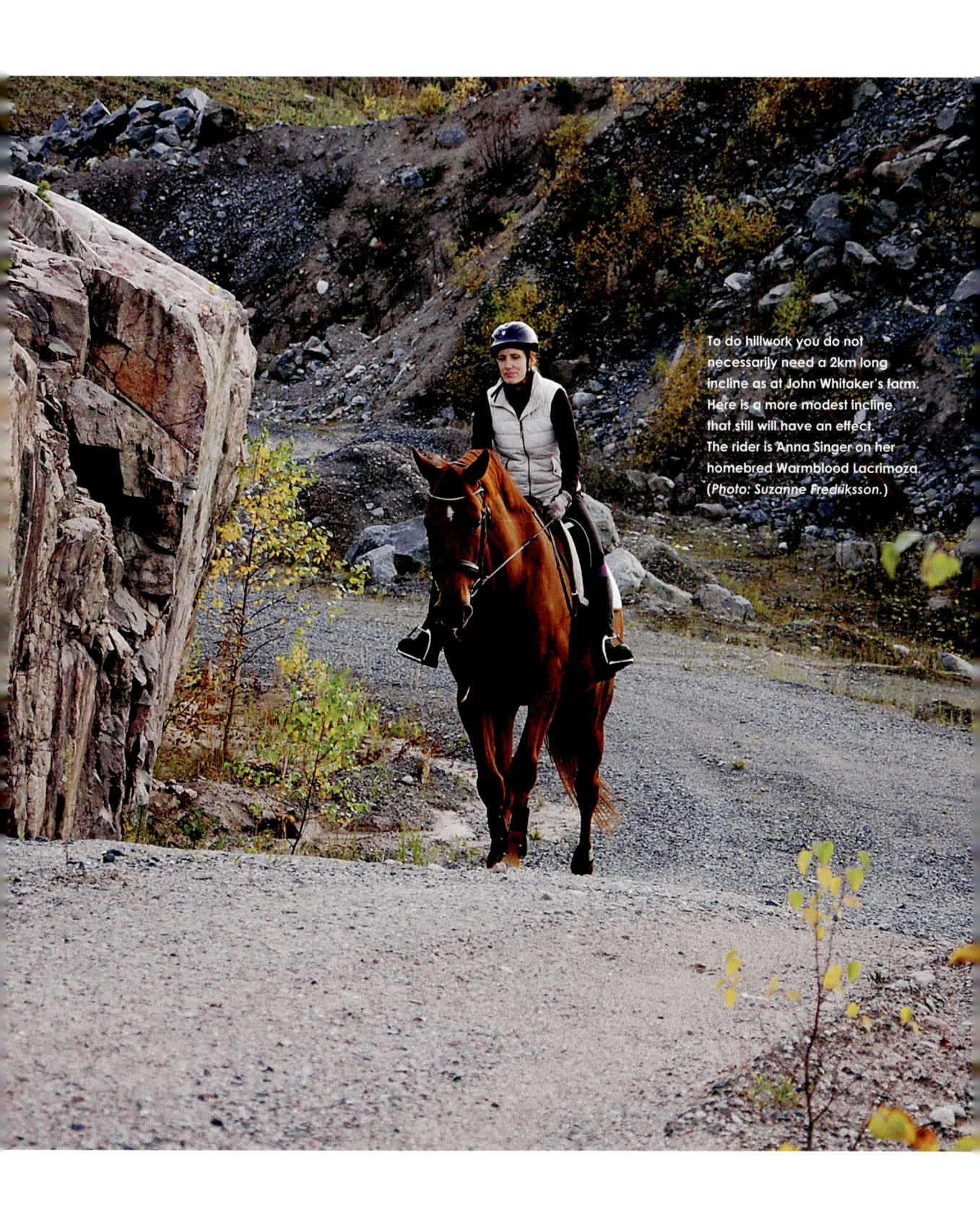

To do hillwork you do not necessarily need a 2km long incline as at John Whitaker's farm. Here is a more modest incline, that still will have an effect. The rider is Anna Singer on her homebred Warmblood Lacrimoza. (Photo: Suzanne Fredriksson.)

Gillian Higgins' book, mentioned in the reading suggestions in Chapter 2, includes exercises on the ground designed to help develop the muscles of the trunk, including the back and tummy. The suggestions are similar as those in a programme developed by Dr Clayton and the Australian equine physio Narelle Stubbs, which are also available in book form (see reading list at the end of Chapter 2). Some experts including Peder Fredricson have the experience that these types of exercises also have a relaxing effect on the horse's mind.

Apart from roadwork, another strong tradition in the British Isles is to use hills and inclines in fitness and strength training. John Whitaker has access to an incline, which means he can ride uphill for 2km in one go. The Dutch study of event horses mentioned earlier found that an incline of ten per cent was sufficient to get an increased training effect, compared to doing the same work on flat ground. When the horse's cardiovascular system and muscles have to work harder because of the incline, rather than because of high speed, you limit the loading on the musculoskeletal system but get a similar training effect. Compare the extra effort involved if you ride a bike or run up just a small hill compared to doing the same thing on a flat road, and how much faster you would have to run or pedal on the flat to get the same effect!

Step 3 – canter/gallop work

Canter or gallop work means cantering/galloping outdoors on a track or very good grass surface. Depending on the speed it can also mean either aerobic work or anaerobic (with lactic acid). Canter work at brisk speeds is the last step in the fitness 'staircase' and should be done only when the horse has first developed a good basic fitness – see phase 1 about roadwork! If you have not done canter work previously, further advice is not to start without supervision and advice from a rider or coach with much more experience.

As we saw earlier, it is important to remember the principle that 'speed kills'. In this context it is normally not the literal case, but the fact that higher speeds do increase the load on bone, joints and tendons and, with that, injury risk. This means that a surface which is even and offers elasticity and suitable grip is very important. In the British Isles and also elsewhere one option is to contact a trainer with private gallops/training tracks, or someone offering gallops, provided they are known for good maintenance.

When you start faster work it is, as with everything else in training, important to start gradually, and with short distances. Both John Whitaker and Dr Hilary Clayton also say that, again, it is important to take into account the individual horse's mental and physical make-up.

Physical training was part of the medal plan

In the run-up to the 2004 Olympics everyone knew that Athens in August would mean hot weather, and therefore extra exertion for the horses. To make sure that the Swedish showjumping team horses had energy to spare the Swedish team 'board' of coach Henk Nooren, chef d'equipe Sylve Söderstrand and team vet Jonas Tornell contacted a top track and field coach to find out more about the training of track and field athletes. They learnt more about anaerobic training and developed a fitness programme for the Swedish Olympic horses. One ingredient was grid jumping, as a version of interval training. Through measuring heart rate and lactic acid levels Dr Tornell found that, with a number of sets of gridwork over smallish fences, you could replicate the level of exertion when jumping a 1.60m course, without the loading of bone, joints and tendons that such big fences normally result in. Sweden won the team silver, after advancing in the last round when other teams faded.

Dr Tornell kept a fitness training programme for the team horses, scheduled for a build-up period in the beginning of the year. It is divided into three phases. In the first the horses do physical training exercises three days a week, all using the interval principle; hillwork, gridwork and canter work. One day a week is a rest day, with only walking and paddock time. Phase 2, from the end of January, include two days a week with grid work and interval/hillwork. From the end of February the horses normally compete more often and then there is only one fitness session per week, with either gridwork or a few high fences.

SPORT HORSE SOUNDNESS AND PERFORMANCE

Research: training strategies
Strategies for showjumping horses

So how is a training programme for successful showjumpers designed? There is really only one study done; the European Footing and Training study we have already mentioned. The findings are also of interest for both dressage and eventing; it is only the proportions of discipline-specific training that will vary – and of course the event horses are alone in training over cross-country fences (although there is tradition that all young horses benefit from an introduction to jumping cross-country, that is supported by some coaches).

The study riders in Sweden, the UK, Switzerland and the Netherlands were at elite level but, as professionals, did not only train horses at S (advanced) level, but also young horses from four years of age. How, and how much, the horses were trained varied significantly between the riders:

■ How many ridden sessions per week (varied from 4.6 to 6.2).
■ How long was the session (varied from 19 to 49 minutes).

The following activities were included in the training plan:

- All riders did **flatwork** (dressage) but how often varied from 1.4 to 4.8 sessions per week.
- How much **hacking** (in the forest, on bridlepaths or fields) the horses did as a percentage of the total training varied from five to 45 per cent, (or from less than one twentieth to almost half of all training time).
- All riders except four **lunged** their horses as part of the training regimen.
- In Sweden, where some speed testing was done, five of the riders did **canter work** slower than 400m per minute. Four of the Swedish riders did canter work on a racing track (for trotting or for other equestrian use) and in one case at up to 700m per minute.
- Five Swedish riders used **hillwork** in their training.
- Additional activities (one or two riders each): **loose jumping**, **loose canters in a arena**, **treadmill work**, **long-reining**.
- Time for non-ridden activities (so how much time daily the horses spent outside the stable) also varied greatly between riders. Including paddock turnout it was from 1.3 to 11.3 hours.
- All riders except one in the four countries **let the horses out in a field/paddock**. The mean daily time was 3.8 hours, but then for some riders double that.
- All riders except one used a **walker** in the daily work.
- All except five **led their horses out in hand** as light exercise or for relaxation, especially at shows.
- The mean percentage of planned rest days was 23 per cent, but varied from ten to 38 per cent. In other words, the average horse had a rest day every fourth day, but some had one every ten days and others almost every second day.

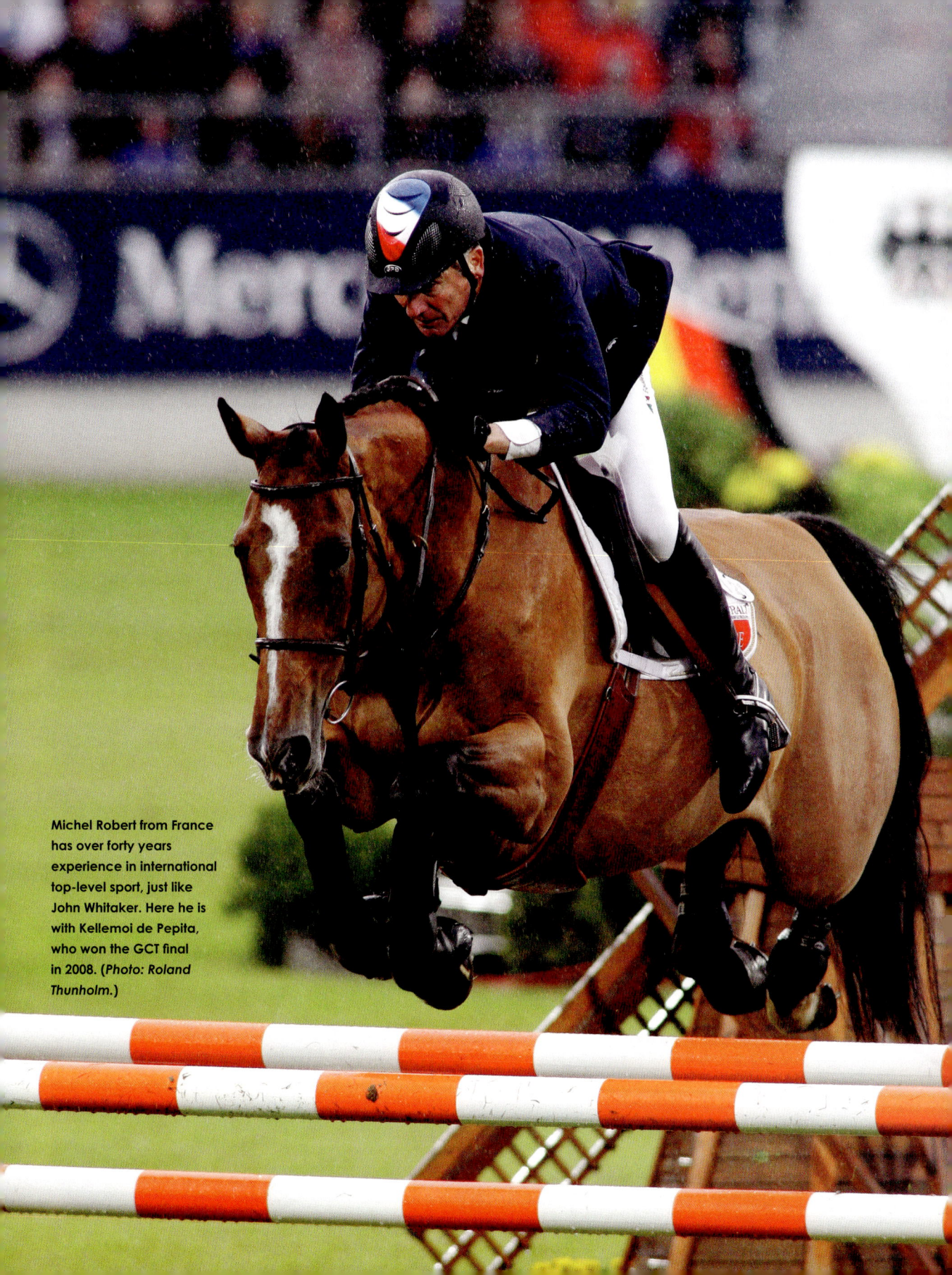

Michel Robert from France has over forty years experience in international top-level sport, just like John Whitaker. Here he is with Kellemoi de Pepita, who won the GCT final in 2008. (*Photo: Roland Thunholm.*)

SPORT HORSE SOUNDNESS AND PERFORMANCE

Research: training strategies
Strategies for dressage horses

The same research group at the Animal Health Trust in England, who showed that horses from different disciplines are more likely to get different injuries (or in different anatomic locations) has also studied the training of dressage horses in relation to injury. They did a postal questionnaire study with some 2,500 members of British Dressage, having first contacted all 20,000 members. The profile of those who replied compared to the majority of BD member is therefore unknown, and the results should therefore be viewed with some reservations, and apply to UK conditions. Still, it gives a valuable insight into dressage training and competition strategies.

- Horses did **on average two shows per month**, except at Grand Prix level, when it was once.

- Most horses spent about **15–30 hours per week in the paddock/field**.

- 95 per cent of the horses had other training than only dressage work in an arena, mainly **hacking** plus, for a smaller percentage, **lungeing and jumping**.

- The horses at Advanced level were, however, a lot less likely to go hacking or jumping.

- The number of **dressage work sessions** was on average three to four per week.

- **Warming up and cooling down** at all levels lasted on average 16 minutes and 11 minutes respectively, and the actual dressage work 36 minutes: 21 per cent walk, 45 per cent trot and 32 per cent canter.

- The exercises included transitions (30–39 per cent), specific movements (30–39 per cent), working trot/canter (40–49 per cent), collection (10–19 per cent) and extensions (0–9 per cent). Not surprisingly, horses at Advanced level did more collected work and less in working trot or canter than those on lower levels.

Ida-Linn Lundholm on the approved KWPN stallion Ampere 1225 preparing for a stallion show at Tullstorp Dressage Stable in southern Sweden. (*Photo: Krister Lindh/Tullstorp.*)

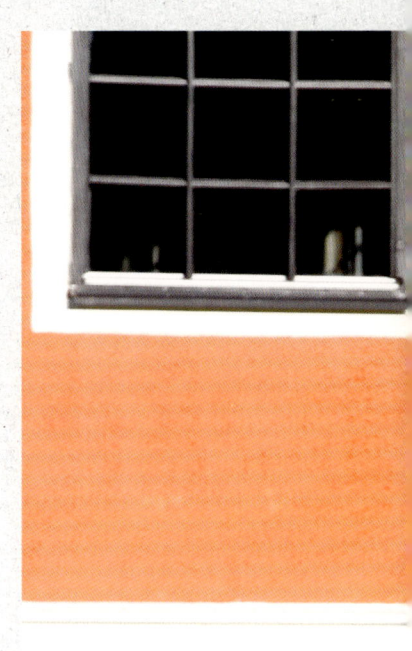

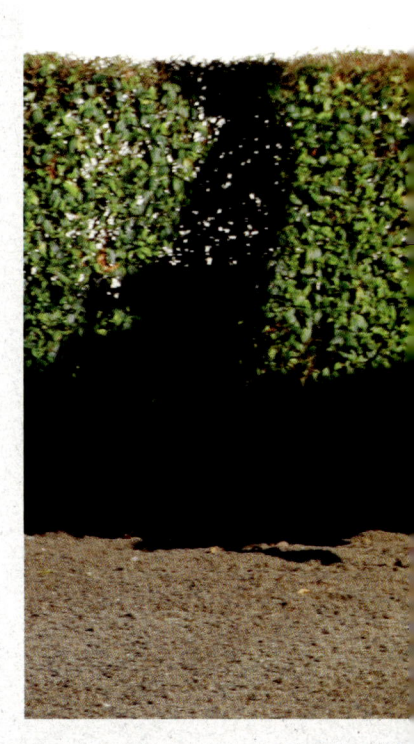

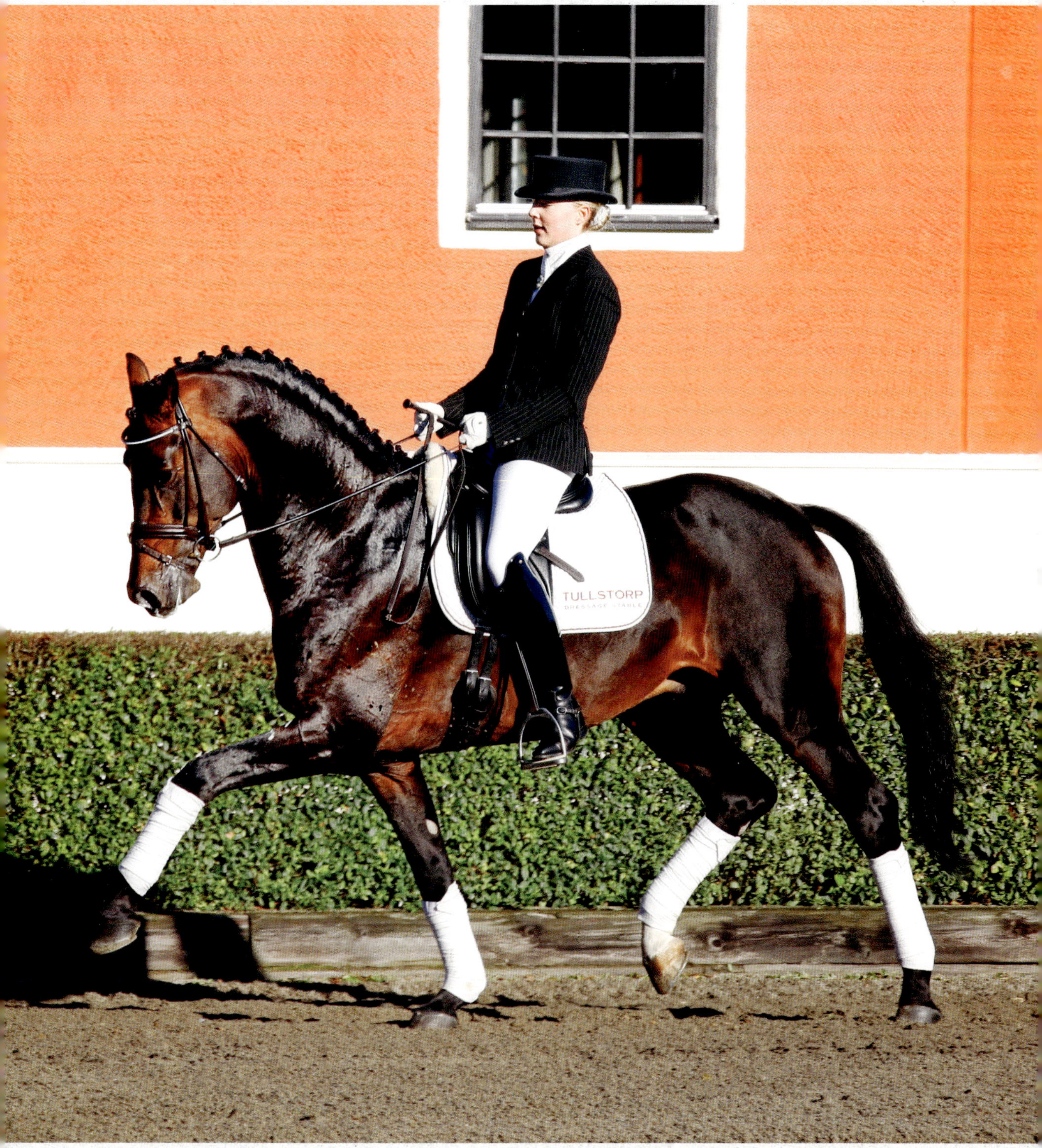
TULLSTORP
DRESSAGE STABLE

10. Competition plans and travel

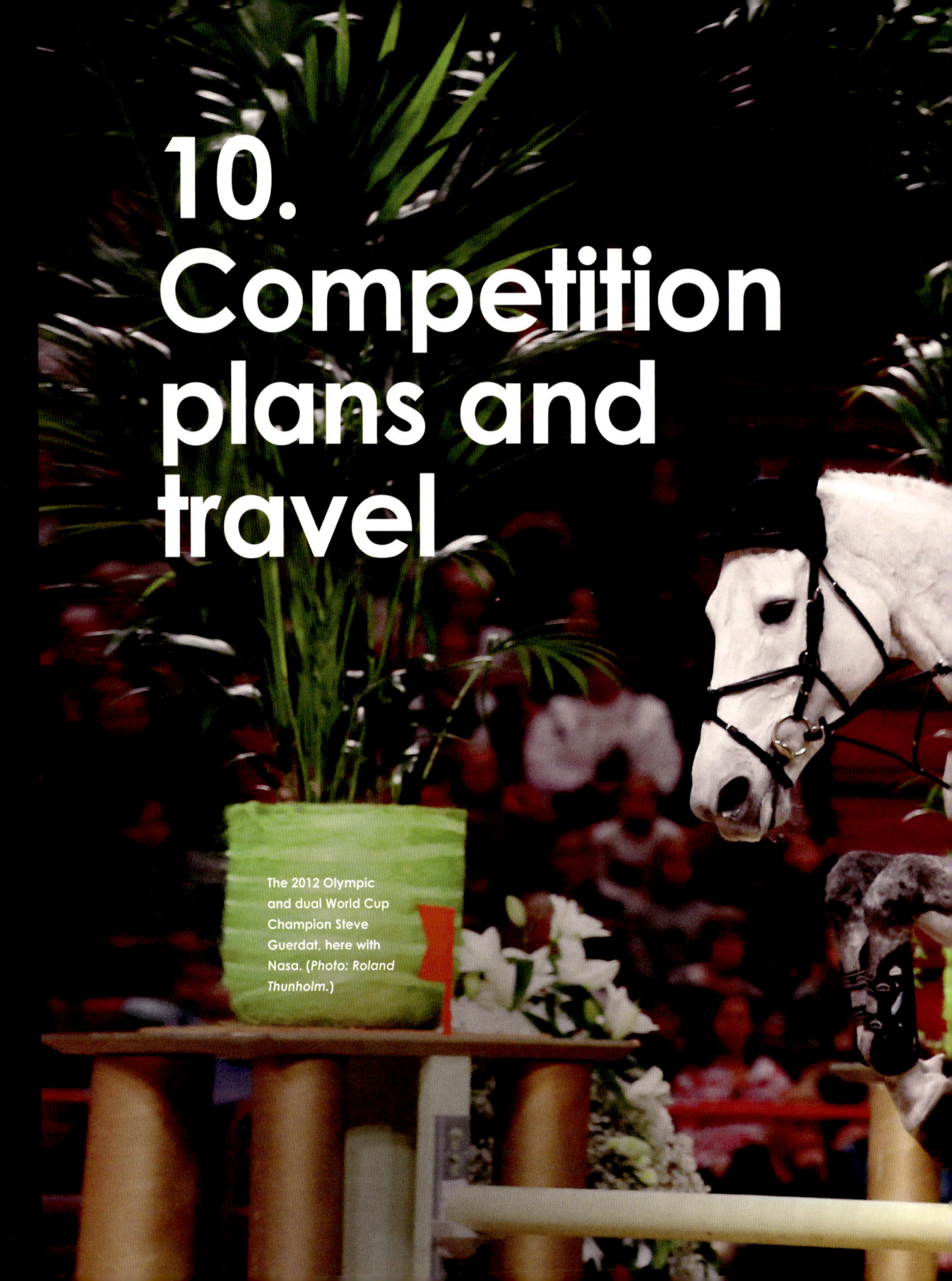

The 2012 Olympic and dual World Cup Champion Steve Guerdat, here with Nasa. (*Photo: Roland Thunholm.*)

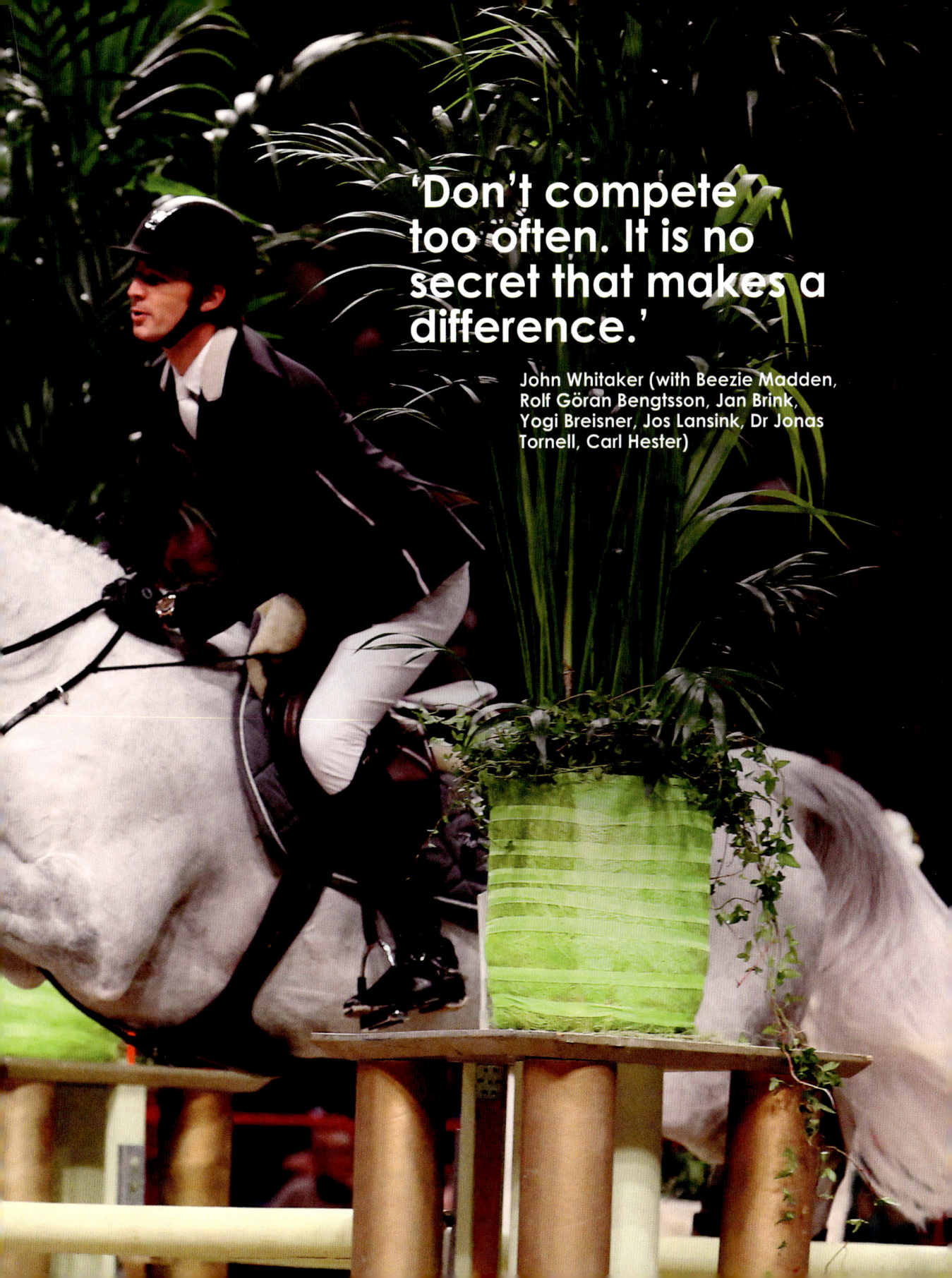

'Don't compete too often. It is no secret that makes a difference.'

John Whitaker (with Beezie Madden, Rolf Göran Bengtsson, Jan Brink, Yogi Breisner, Jos Lansink, Dr Jonas Tornell, Carl Hester)

COMPETITION PLANNING

Plan your competitions carefully and give the horse breaks in between. This is one of the most frequent pieces of advice from champion riders and top vets on prevention of injury. Planned breaks from competition also fits with the principle of rest and recovery in previous chapters. If you want to prevent new injuries or avoid recurrence of an old problem it is important to ration and reflect on:

1. How much jumping the horse does (or dressage work at competition level).

2. What shows are the most important in the year and aim to peak for them, rather than competing year round.

'The problem is that people want to compete every week, but horses are not machines. With a car you can change tyres if one gets worn out, but that is impossible with a horse. You must respect the horse and choose your competitions carefully. It is important to have a plan for the season and the horse, and to have a specific aim for that season', Jos Lansink said.

'Make a sensible competition plan, over time and for each show. One example is that you not necessarily try to win the Friday class if you are doing the Grand Prix on the Sunday. It is a question of management', Rolf Göran Bengtsson said.

'Ration your jumping. Do not compete too much. It is no secret that makes a difference', John Whitaker said.

'We ration our competitions. Our horses seldom do more than two or three starts in a week, and they seldom do more than two weeks in a row. At the end of the year they get a complete rest from competition, without shoes and with lots of paddock time for six to eight weeks, so that they get to "be a horse" and relax', Beezie Madden said.

'When you have planned your competitions, make a point of still listening to the horse and skip one or more shows if the horse feels off-colour. If you push on in spite of the horse not being 100 per cent the big problem injuries occur', Jan Brink said.

> An Italian study, measuring muscle response to showjumpers in competition, indicated that five days recovery period between two consecutive competitions is insufficient to allow muscle recovery and avoid potential additional stress.

How many shows?

If you are a showjumper planning your competition schedule, it is valuable to reflect and calculate the workload in competition for a showjumping horse: 18–20 competitions per year with two to three classes per show makes up to 60 starts in total (plus any jump-offs). This can translate into some 1,200 jumping efforts. That is in the arena, not counting the warm-up. If the rider does in addition 15–25 warm-up jumps per class in three starts that adds up to 75 jumps per show, and 1,500 jumps per year. So a horse doing 20 shows in a year with three classes each would jump some 2,700 times just at shows, not counting in training. Doing just a few more practice jumps before each class, and/or competing at a few more shows could add around 1,000 more jumping efforts per year. Veterinary comment is that some champion riders (who confirm this themselves) restrict their warm-up jumps to about 15 per class.

Warming up is important but, because it adds to overall effort, the guidelines offered by experienced sport horse vets are that, at international level, horses should be doing a maximum of 15–17 showjumping competitions a year, and six to eight dressage competitions. At international level the intensity of the calendar means that many horses do more, but how that translates into length of competition career is worth pondering. As late as the 1970s the international show calendar ended in late autumn and only started in February-March, giving horses a natural winter break.

Carl Hester has explained the strategy for Valegro during most of his international career as planning the season based on that year's international championship and doing only about two or three other shows, as he performed at his best when fresh and did not need practice.

Peaking and tapering

This is an expression in sports training which is very similar to when top riders talk of their planning for important goals such as championships. 'Peaking' means reaching the top of your form at pre-selected time slots and 'tapering' is having a 'breather' ahead of that, simply put, in order to store energy. One important principle is, then, as Carl Hester and many other champion riders mention, to determine early which are the most important shows of the year and to plan the season accordingly. In the run-up to an important show the horse should be allowed to 'load the battery' and not compete except lightly.

Annual holiday

Several of the riders quoted in this book give their horses an annual holiday, especially in the winter. For example Beezie Madden and Pippa Funnell let their horses out in fields, without shoes, to 'be horses' for about two months – the equivalent of summer pasture for the riding school horses. Other riders let their horses have winter or other breaks with relaxation and some light exercise, but not just standing still in the stable or in a small paddock.

TRAVELLING (TO COMPETITIONS)

As a rider, you want to optimise your horse's chances of performing at his best. One important factor is to make sure that travelling to and from competitions is as comfortable and undemanding as possible. How well the horse travels, how far, and ensuring that he drinks sufficiently and does not lose fluids, are very important factors that can affect performance. This was pointed out both by specialists at the EEHNC in 2015 and by Franke Sloothaak:

'In the beginning, travelling is something that the horses need to be allowed to get used to and learn. It is, of course, a novelty for a horse who has only been away for a day when he is staying overnight in a different stable for the first time', Sloothaak said.

Here is some expert advice on horse travel. (It is, of course, valid also for transporting horses not involved in competitions. Several of the points are from research studies, but are also based on practical experience and were presented at the EEHNC and by Dr Philippe Benoit at CESMAS (Conference on Equine Sports Medicine and Science) in 2010.

- Horses should always be transported as comfortably and as relaxed as possible, to preserve energy for the show.
- Air quality in the transport, the driver's style of driving and the type of transport will influence the aims just mentioned. Ensuring that the horse travels in comfort can be expensive, but is important. How the horse needs to balance himself in the lorry or trailer will affect how tiring the journey will be for him, Benoit said.
- Include the travel time to and from shows when you do your competition plans – take into account how long the journey is when you estimate the total effort for the horse during a competition weekend.
- The driving style can have a major effect on how comfortable or uncomfortable the horse is during the trip, so pay attention to how you, or anyone else, are driving.
- Make stops during the trip, and respect rules on maximum transport hours.

SPORT HORSE SOUNDNESS AND PERFORMANCE

- It is important that the horse is positioned in a way that he can lower his head to the ground. This helps prevent respiratory infection and with that travel sickness.
- Water! It is very important to supervise the horse's water intake during the journey and make sure he is drinking properly, to avoid dehydration. The same is valid at shows, especially in hot weather. A correct fluid balance in the body is vital for performance and well-being. Even a low degree of dehydration can result in the horse entering a viscous (and dangerous) cycle when he stops drinking. This can also increase the risk of transport sickness and of impaction colic.

Flying is a routine matter for today's top international showjumpers.
(Photo: Roland Thunholm.)

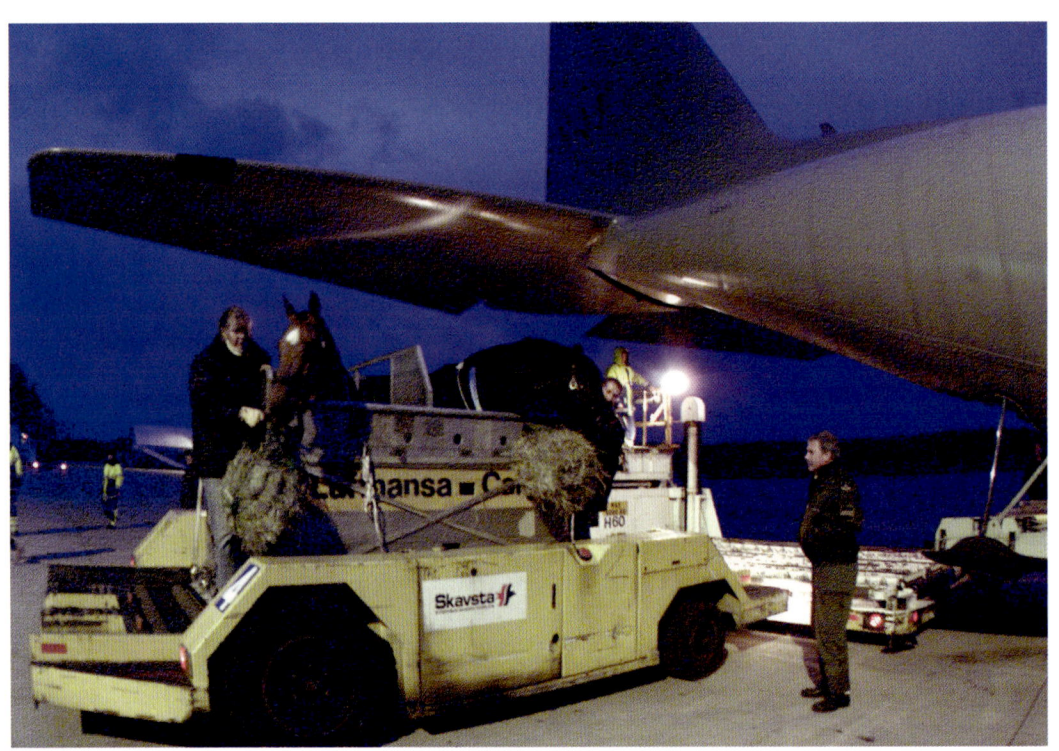

Jumping megastar Ludger Beerbaum also mentions the importance of water in his bullet point advice in Chapter 3.

This consideration was also stressed at the EEHNC, when the theme was looking after the sport horse. Many riders and grooms pay attention to giving the horse electrolytes, but if, at the same time, he does not drink sufficiently it will not help the fluid balance at all, the French endurance team vet Celine Robert said at the Congress.

Advice about fluids and water

1. Measure at home how much the horse drinks during an ordinary day, and you can then use that to compare with consumption at a show, Anky van Grunsven pointed out at the EEHNC. Measure his water consumption from a bucket. (There is a Swedish study showing that how the horse is offered water – from a bucket or from an automatic drinker – will affect how much he drinks, and the flow in an automatic drinker is not always enough).
2. Test at home what might tempt the horse to drink a bit more, for example if he likes the taste of water with some apple juice, that will disguise if the water has a different taste at a show.
3. Two buckets, one with ordinary water and one with some extra good taste added, is another suggestion, as some horses do not like drinking all the water in one bucket, but rather drinks half each of two buckets. This suggestion comes from the Belgian eventing veteran Karen Donckers, who was sixth at the 2016 World Equestrian Games.
4. A fourth tip is to bring the horse's everyday bucket from home, so that the smell seems familiar.
5. On longer journeys: be vigilant for any signs of transport sickness (fever, listlessness, less appetite).

SPORT HORSE SOUNDNESS AND PERFORMANCE

Avoid ferries!

To save road distance by taking a ferry with the horse lorry or trailer can appear to be a smooth way to travel. But those with plenty of experience avoid ferry trips if there is a road alternative, or take the shortest possible route if a land route is not feasible. This is because ferry trips appear to increase the risk of the horse contracting travel sickness owing to poor air quality down on a car deck. Another problem on a ferry is that there is no option to get off or stop if the horse has a problem, and you will not be allowed on in windy weather. Aeroplanes you cannot get off either, but they seem to offer smoother travel than a boat, provided that an experienced equine transport company is in charge.

Former World Champion Jos Lansink and the stallion Spender S at home. (Photo: Roland Thunholm.)

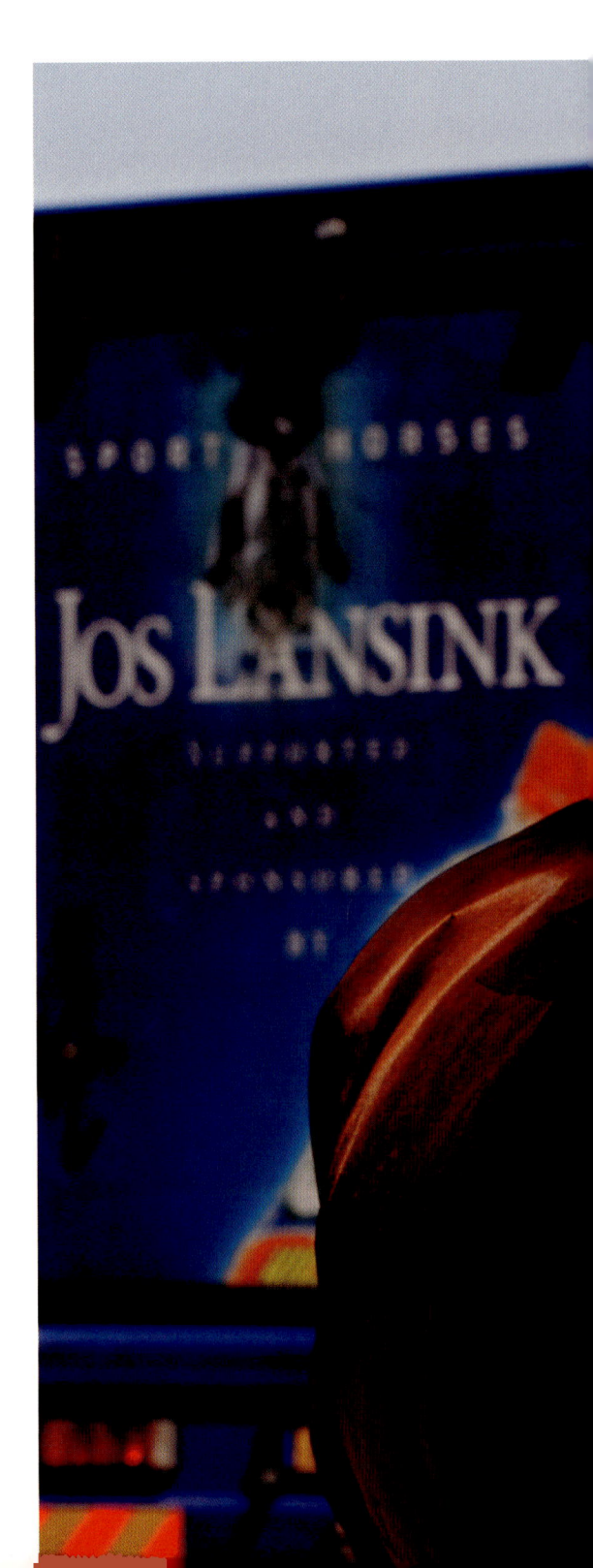

COMPETITION PLANS AND TRAVEL

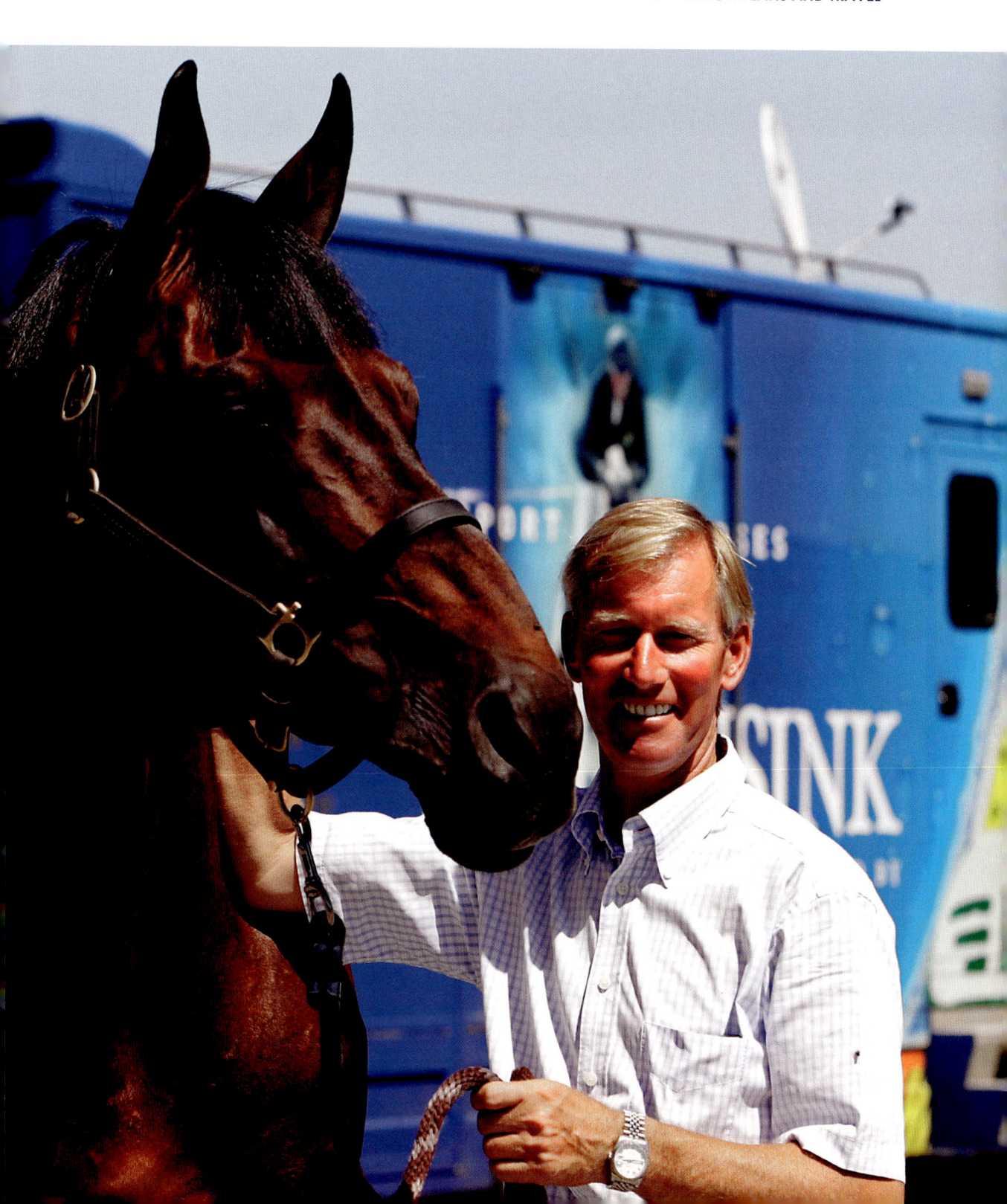

11. Supplements, medication and doping

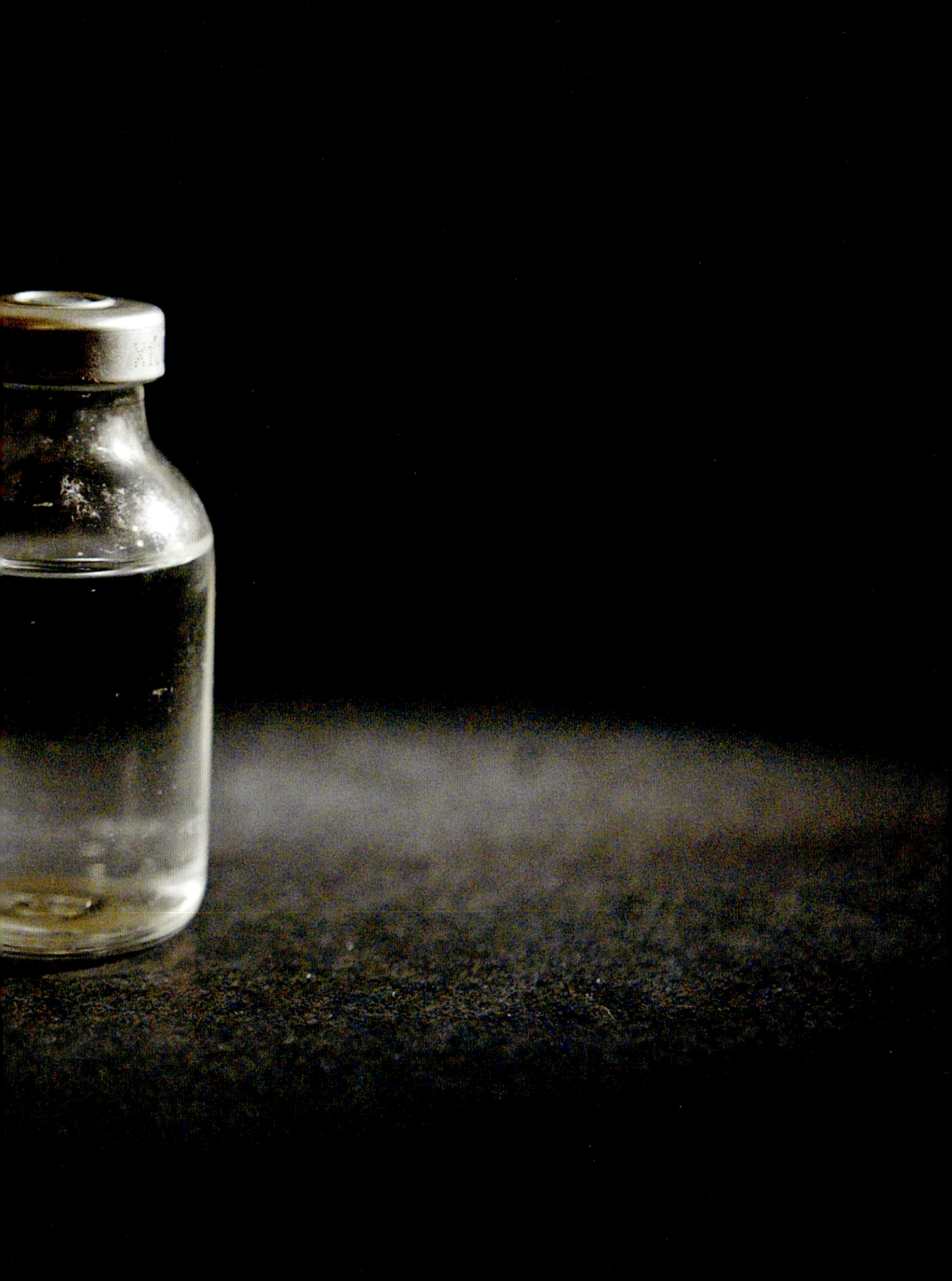

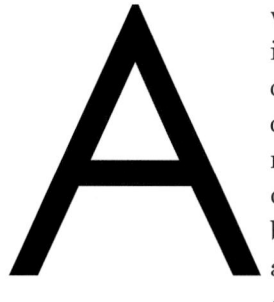

A whole riding career, or at least the most important competition in your life, can be spoilt by a doping/medication case. There are examples both at national and international level of disqualifications and bans arising from both conscious, but misguided, actions and genuine mistakes by, for example, a groom or a friend.

There is a crucial difference between anti-doping rules for horses versus human athletes. When equine cases occur they are often discussed as 'doping', but it is important to realise that, for horses, almost all substances are banned in connection with competitions and races! So a number of famous human athletes who won titles while on painkillers would have been disqualified if they were horses. Many riders have made the mistake of thinking equine anti-doping rules concern only performance-enhancing substances, which is a general principle in human sports. But in horse sports, or at least those presided over by the International Equestrian Federation, European equestrian federations and many (but not all) racing jurisdictions, basically all medications are banned before and during competitions. The background is the view that the horse should be protected from competing with, for example, an injury or sickness masked by medication, while human athletes are free to make that risk analysis themselves.

The rules today for sport horses differ between positive cases of:

Doping: administration of prohibited substances that can affect performance and/or have such properties, including side-effects, that they should never be given to horses anyway. Cases can result in several years ban, plus fines.

Controlled medication: administration of drugs that are

References – scientific studies

A key focus of the book is quotes from scientific research. The major ones are listed below. What defines a scientific article are that the design, results and conclusions have been reviewed and approved by other experts in the same field prior to publishing. The list shows the names of the scientists who conducted the study, the title (which often describes something about the results in just a few words), the year of publication, and the scientific journal where it was published, with page numbers. Some references are given as background to illustrate research in the field, others are directly quoted in the text.

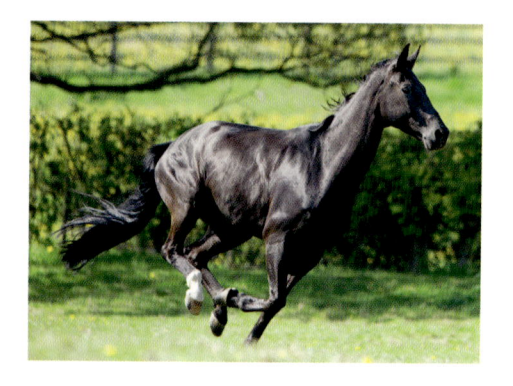

Chapter 1
Background – why this book?

Egenvall A., Lönnell C., Roepstorff L., 'Analysis of morbidity and mortality data in riding school horses, with special regard to locomotor problems' (March 2009), *Preventive Veterinary Medicine,* Vol 88 (3): 193–204.

Egenvall A., Tranquille C., Lönnell C., Bitschnau C., Oomen A., Hernlund E., Montavon S., Franko M., Murray R., Weishaupt M., van Weeren R., Roepstorff L., 'Days lost to training and competition in relation to workload in 263 elite showjumping horses in four European countries' (November 2013), *Preventive Veterinary Medicine,* Vol 112 (3–4): 387–400.

Rossdale P.D., Hopes R., Digby N.J., Offord K., 'Epidemiological study of wastage among racehorses 1982 and 1983' (January 1985), *Veterinary Record,* Vol 116 (3): 66–9.

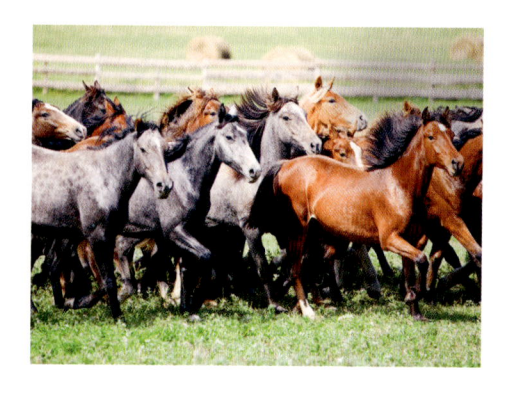

Chapter 2
The horse's body

Egenvall A., Penell J.C., Bonnett B.N., Olson P., Pringle J., 'Mortality of Swedish horses with complete life insurance between 1997 and 2000: variations with sex, age, breed and diagnosis (March 2006), *Veterinary Record,* Vol 158 (12): 397–406.

Chapter 3
Preventing injury

Dyson P.K., Jackson B.F., Pfeiffer D.U., Price J.S., 'Days lost to training by two- and three-year-old Thoroughbred horses: A survey of seven UK training yards' (November 2008), *Equine Veterinary Journal,* Vol 40 (7): 650–7.

Estberg L., Gardner I.A., Stover S.M., Johnson B.J., Case J.T., Ardans A., 'Cumulative racing-speed exercise distance cluster as a risk factor for fatal musculoskeletal injury in Thoroughbred racehorses in California' (October 1995), *Preventive Veterinary Medicine,* Vol 24 (4): 253–63.

Munsters C.B.M., van den Broek J., Welling E., van Weeren R., Sloet van Oldruitenborgh-Oosterbaan M., 'A prospective study on a cohort of horses and ponies selected for participation in the European Eventing Championship: reasons for withdrawal and predictive value of fitness tests' (September 2013), *BMC Veterinary Research,* Vol 9: 182.

Murray R.C., Dyson S.J., Tranquille C., Adams V., 'Association of type of sport and performance level with anatomical site of orthopaedic injury diagnosis' (August 2006), *Equine Veterinary Journal,* Vol 38 (S36): 411–16.

Murray R.C., Walters J.M., Snart H., Dyson S.J., Parkin T.D., 'Identification of risk factors for lameness in dressage horses' (April 2010), *The Veterinary Journal,* Vol 184 (1): 27–36.

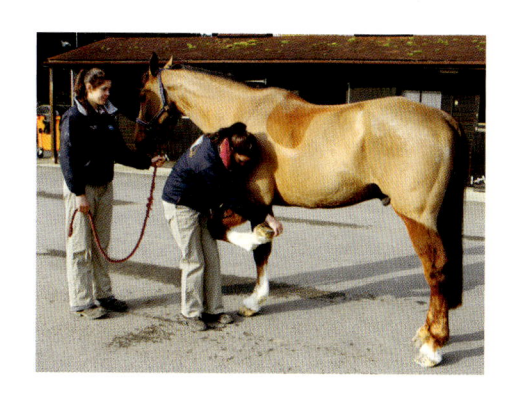

O'Brien E., Stevens KB., Pfeiffer DU., Hall J., Marr CM., 'Factors associated with the wastage and achievements in competition of event horses registered in the United Kingdom' (July 2005), *Veterinary Record,* Vol 157 (1): 9–13.

Reed S.R., Jackson B., McIlwraith C.W., Wright I.M., Pilsworth R., Knapp S., Wood J.L.N., Price J.S., Verheyen K.L.P., 'Descriptive epidemiology of joint injuries in Thoroughbred racehorses in training' (January 2012), *Equine Veterinary Journal,* Vol 44 (1): 13–19.

Reed R., Jackson B.,Wood J., Price J., Verheyen K., 'Exercise affects joint injury risk in young Thoroughbreds in training' (June 2013), *The Veterinary Journal,* Vol 196 (3): 339–344.

Singer E.R., Barnes J., Saxby F., Murray J.K., 'Injuries in the event horse: Training versus competition' (January 2008), *The Veterinary Journal,* Vol 175 (1): 76–81.

Parkin T.D.H., Clegg P.D., French N.P., Proudman C.J., Riggs C.M., Singer E.R., Webbon P.M., Morgan K.L., 'Horse level risk factors for fatal distal limb fracture in racing Thoroughbreds in the UK' (September 2004), *Equine Veterinary Journal,* Vol 36 (6): 513–19.

Verheyen K.L., Price J.S., Lanyon L., Wood J., 'Exercise distance and speed affect the risk of fracture in racehorses' (December 2006), *Bone,* Vol 39 (1): 1322–30.

Chapter 4
The 'right' horse – are you a good match?

Cornelissen B.P., van Weeren P.R., Ederveen A.G., Barneveld A., 'Influence of exercise on bone mineral density of immature cortical and trabecular bone of the equine metacarpus and proximal sesamoid bone' (November 1999), *Equine Veterinary Journal,* Vol 31 (S31): 79–85.

Diesterbeck U.S., Hertsch B., Distl O., 'Genome-wide search for microsatellite markers associated with radiologic alterations in the navicular bone of Hannoverian warmblood horses' (May 2007), *Mammalian Genome,* Vol 18 (5): 373–81.

Wallin L., Strandberg E., Philipsson J., Dalin G., 'Estimates of longevity and causes of culling and death in Swedish warmblood and coldblood horses' (May 2000), *Livestock Production Science,* Vol 63 (1): 275–89.

Weller R., Pfau T., Verheyen K., May S.A., Wilson A.M., 'The effect of conformation on orthopaedic health and performance in a cohort of National Hunt racehorses: preliminary results' (November 2006), *Equine Veterinary Journal,* Vol 38 (7): 622–7.

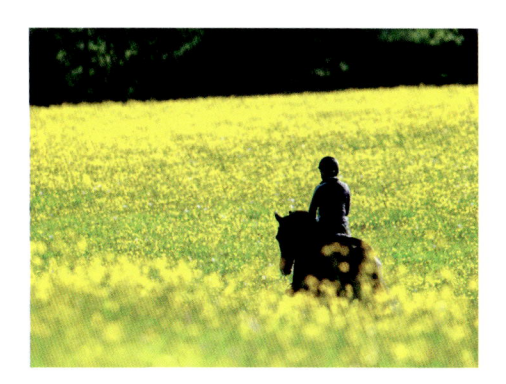

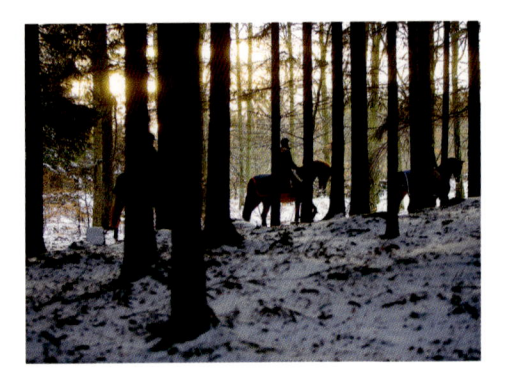

Chapter 5
Allow your horse time

Lönnell C., Roepstorff L., Egenvall A., 'Variation in equine management factors between riding schools with high vs. low insurance claims for orthopaedic injury: a field study' (July 2012), *The Veterinary Journal,* Vol 193 (1): 109–13.

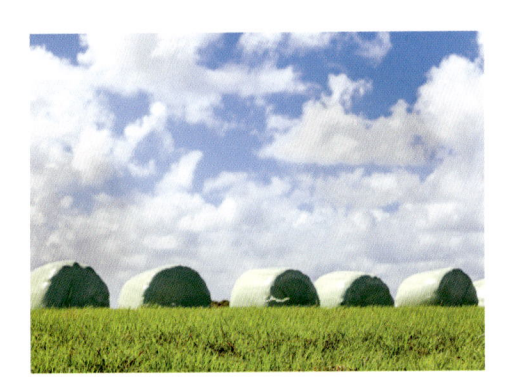

Chapter 7
Feeding, supplements and water

Oke S., Aghazadeh-Habashi A., Weese J.S, Jamali S., 'Evaluation of glucosamine levels in commercial equine oral supplements for joints' (January 2006), *Equine Veterinary Journal,* Vol 38 (1) 93–95.

Ringmark S., Roepstorff L., Essén-Gustavsson B., Revold T., Lindholm A., Hedenström U., Rundgren M., Ögren G., Jansson A., 'Growth, training response and health in Standardbred yearlings fed a forage-only diet' (May 2013), *Animal,* Vol 7 (5): 746–53.

Chapter 8
Riding surfaces – vary where you ride

Hernlund E., Egenvall A., Peterson M., Mahaffey C., Roepstorff L., 'Hoof accelerations at hoof-surface impact for stride types and functional limb types relevant to showjumping horses' (December 2013), *The Veterinary Journal,* Vol 198 (1): e27–e32.

Peterson M., McIlwraith CW., Reiser II RF. 'Development of a system for the *in-situ* characterisation of Thoroughbred horse racing track surfaces' (October 2008), *Biosystems Engineering,* Vol 101 (2): 260–9.

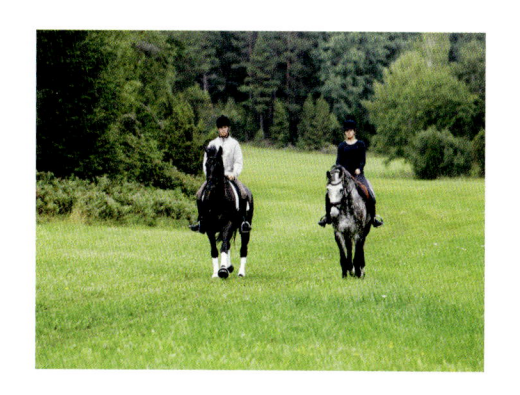

Chapter 9
Training

Braam A., Nasholm A., Roepstorff L., Philipsson J., 'Genetic variation in durability of Swedish Warmblood horses using competition results' (December 2011), *Livestock Science,* Vol 142 (1–3): 181–7.

Docking SI., Daffy J., van Schie HTM., Cook JL., 'Tendon structure changes after maximal exercise in the Thoroughbred horse: use of ultrasound tissue characterization to detect in vivo tendon response' (December 2012), *The Veterinary Journal,* Vol 194 (3): 338–342.

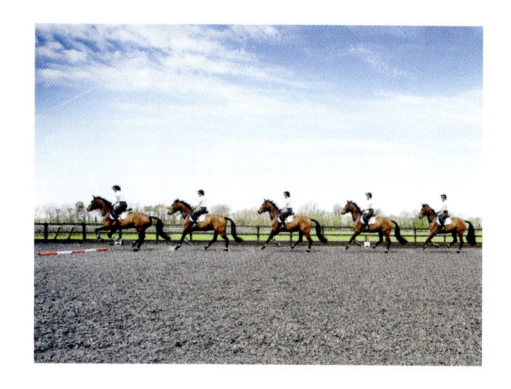

Hampson B.A., Morton J.M., Mills P.C., Travter M.G., Lamb D.W., Pollitt C.C., 'Monitoring distances travelled by horses using GPS tracking collars' (April 2010), *Australian Veterinary Journal,* Vol 88 (5): 176–81.

Lönnell C., Bröjer J., Nostell K., Hernlund E., Roepstorff L., Tranquille C., Murray R., Oomen A., van Weeren R., Bitschnau C., Montavon S., Weishaupt M., Egenvall A., 'Variations in training regimens in professional showjumping yards' (March 2014), *Equine Veterinary Journal,* Vol 46 (2): 233–8.

Murray R., Mann C., Parkin T., 'Warm-up in dressage competitions: association with level, competition type and final score' (November 2006), *Equine and Comparative Exercise Physiology,* Vol 3 (4): 185–9.

Tranquille C., Walker V., Hodgins D., Goosen T., McEwen J., 'Quantifying warm-up in showjumping horses over 3 consecutive days' (June 2014), *Equine Veterinary Journal*, Vol 46 (S46): 10–11.

Uemura Y., Ishiko T., Yamauchi T., Kurono M., Mashiko S., 'Five jumps per day increase bone mass and breaking force in rats' (September 1997), *Journal of Bone and Mineral Research*, Vol 12 (9): 1480–5.

Walker V; Walters J., Griffith L., Murray R., 'The effect of collection and extension on tarsal flexion and fetlock extension at trot' (March 2013) *Equine Veterinary Journal,* Vol 45 (2): 245–8.

Walters J., Parkin T., Snart H.A., Murray R.C., 'Current management and training practices for UK dressage horses' (May 2008), *Comparative Exercise Physiology,* Vol 5 (2): 73–83.

Chapter 10
Competition plans and travel

Assenza A., Marafioti S., Congiu F., Giannetto C., Fazio F., Bruschetta D., Piccione G., 'Serum muscle-derived enzymes response during show jumping competition in horse' (March 2016) *Veterinary World,* Vol 9 (3): 251–5.

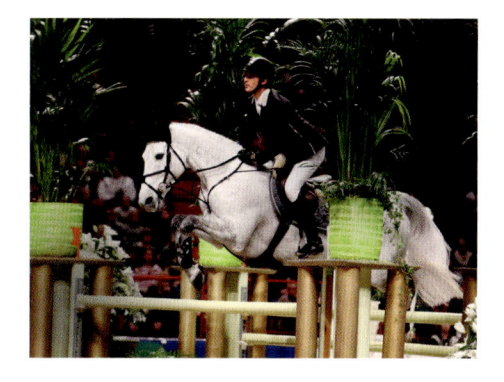